Official Journal of the International Society for Neuroimmunomodulation

NeuroImmunoModulation

Founded 1994 by S.M. McCann and J.M. Lipton
Continued by G.P. Chrousos (2002–2006)

KARGER

Printed in Switzerland on acid-free and non-aging paper (ISO 9706) by Reinhardt Druck, Basel

Appears bimonthly: 1 volume per year (6 issues)

Guidelines for Authors

NeuroImmunoModulation

Aims and Scope

The rapidly expanding area of research known as neuroimmunomodulation explores the way in which the nervous system interacts with the immune system via neural, hormonal, and paracrine actions. Encompassing both basic and clinical research, 'Neuroimmunomodulation' reports on all aspects of these interactions. Basic investigations consider all neural and humoral interactions from molecular genetics through cell regulation to integrative systems of the body. The journal also aims to clarify the basic mechanisms involved in the pathogenesis of the CNS pathology in AIDS patients and in various neurodegenerative diseases. Although primarily devoted to research articles, timely reviews will be published on a regular basis. To ensure high quality, all papers will be reviewed by at least two referees, with every effort made to maintain a short publication time.

Manuscripts

should be submitted using the online submission website at:

www.karger.com/nim

Authors are asked to suggest three to four potential reviewers for their manuscript. These experts on the topic of the article should not be from the same institution as the author(s). The names and the full postal and e-mail addresses of potential reviewers should be submitted with each article. Editors will consider these suggestions but are not bound by them.

Should you experience any problems with your submission, please contact the Editorial Office:

nim@karger.ch

Conditions

All manuscripts are subject to editorial review. Manuscripts are received with the explicit understanding that they are not under simultaneous consideration by any other publication. Submission of an article for publication implies the transfer of the copyright from the author to the publisher upon acceptance. Accepted papers become the permanent property of 'Neuroimmunomodulation' and may not be reproduced by any means, in whole or in part, without the written consent of the publisher. It is the author's responsibility to obtain permission to reproduce illustrations, tables, etc. from other publications.

Most reviews are solicited by the editors. Unsolicited reviews may also be considered, but authors should send a brief proposal to the editorial office, summarizing the topic of the proposed review and 4–5 key references.

Manuscripts should be written in English. They should contain unpublished results of research work, and should be as concise as possible. They should be typewritten on 'letter-quality' paper printed on one side of the sheet only and double spaced with a wide margin. Please send the original and three first-class copies of the manuscript. One set of the original illustrations plus three copies is adequate, except in the case of photomicrographs or other illustrations that do not reproduce well in Xerox or related types of copying equipment. In these instances, it will be necessary to submit four clear prints of each illustration for distribution to the reviewers. The final version of your manuscript and illustrations should be submitted on disk. For details refer to 'Disk Submission' or www.karger.com/journals/disksub.htm. Editorial review and copyediting will be executed from the disk version of your manuscript. The following presentation is recommended: Abstract, Introductory statement on the purpose of the studies, Materials and Methods, Results, Discussion, and References. Commonly accepted abbreviations (e.g. ACTH, TSH, DNA) may be used throughout the text and tables, but a definition should be provided the first time each abbreviation is used. Please limit abbreviations to those in common use, and avoid other abbreviations and acronyms. Contributions will generally be printed in order of acceptance for publication. Contributors should know that one of the criteria considered in reviewing manuscripts is the humane and proper treatment of animals. The editors realize that the use of anesthetics, analgesics, and tranquilizers would defeat the purpose of some experiments. However, the use of painful or otherwise noxious stimuli must be carefully and thoroughly justified in the paper. Papers that do not meet these criteria will not be accepted for publication.

Rapid communications: Manuscripts intended for rapid communication must present new findings of sufficient importance to justify their accelerated appearance. Double-spaced manuscripts cannot exceed 7 pages, including figures, tables and references; longer manuscripts will be returned. Rapid communications are subject to the usual editorial review and are published within 2 months following acceptance. Proofs are sent to the Editors and to the authors.

Arrangement

All pages should be numbered consecutively and carry the author's name in the upper right corner.

Title page: The first page of each paper should carry the title, the authors' full first and last names, and the name of the institute or department where the authors conducted their research work. In addition, the following should be put on the title page: 1. A short title for use as a running head; 2. A list of 3–9 key words for indexing purposes; 3. The name and complete mailing address, phone and fax numbers as well as e-mail address of the individual to whom correspondence, proofs, and requests for reprints should be addressed.

***Abstract:* Each paper needs an abstract of up to 250 words. Abstracts for Original Papers should be structured with subheadings as follows: Objective(s), Methods, Results, Conclusion(s). The words used in the subheadings of the Abstract are not included in the 250 words of the Abstract.**

Footnotes: Avoid footnotes if at all possible. When essential, they should be numbered consecutively and typed at the foot of the appropriate page.

Tables and illustrations: Tables (numbered in arabic numerals) should be prepared on separate sheets, and each should have a suitable heading. Illustrations should be numbered in Arabic numerals and legends for the figures should be submitted on a separate page. For the reproduction of illustrations, only good drawings and original photographs can be accepted; negatives or photocopies cannot be used. Due to technical reasons, figures with a screen background should not be submitted. When possible, group several illustrations on one block for reproduction (max. size 180 × 223 mm) or provide crop marks. On the back of each illustration, indicate its number, the author's name, and 'top' with a soft pencil. Electronically submitted b/w half-tone and color illustrations must have a final resolution of 300 dpi after scaling, line drawings one of 800–1200 dpi.

Color illustrations

Online edition: Color illustrations are reproduced free of charge. In the print version, the illustrations are reproduced in black and white. Please avoid referring to the colors in the text and figure legends.

Print edition: Up to 6 color illustrations per page can be integrated within the text at CHF 760.– per page.

Acknowledgments, including, where relevant, credit to the sources of grant support, should be placed before the references.

References: In the text identify references by Arabic numerals [in square brackets]. Material submitted for publication but not yet accepted should be noted as 'unpublished data' and not be included in the reference list. The list of references should include only those publications which are cited in the text. Do not alphabetize; number references in the order in which they are first mentioned in the text. The surnames of all the authors followed by initials should be given. There should be no punctuation other than a comma to separate the authors. Preferably, please cite all authors. Abbreviate journal names according to the Index Medicus system. (Also see International Committee of Medical Journal Editors: Uniform requirements for manuscripts submitted to biomedical journals. N Engl J Med 1997;336:309–315.)

Examples

(a) Papers published in periodicals: Sun J, Koto H, Chung KF: Interaction of ozone and allergen challenges on bronchial responsiveness and inflammation in sensitised guinea pigs. Int Arch Allergy Immunol 1997;112:191–195.

(b) Papers published only with DOI numbers:
Theoharides TC, Boucher W, Spear K: Serum interleukin-6 reflects disease severity and osteoporosis in mastocytosis patients. Int Arch Allergy Immunol DOI: 10.1159/000063858.

(c) Monographs: Matthews DE, Farewell VT: Using and Understanding Medical Statistics, ed 3, revised. Basel, Karger, 1996.

(d) Edited books: Parren PWHI, Burton DR: Antibodies against HIV-1 from phage display libraries: Mapping of an immune response and progress towards antiviral immunotherapy; in Capra JD (ed): Antibody Engineering. Chem Immunol. Basel, Karger, 1997, vol 65, pp 18–56.

(e) Papers published in electronic format: Black CA: Delayed type hypersensitivity: Current theories with a historic perspective. Dermatol Online J 1999;5:7. http://dermatology.cdlib.org/DOJvol5num1.

Papers that have been submitted to a journal but are not yet accepted should not be listed in the bibliography, but the data in them can be referred to in the text as unpublished observations. If details of methods are only available in papers that are 'in press', copies of the papers should be included with the manuscript submitted to 'Neuroimmunomodulation', so that the editorial referees can have adequate information to judge the manuscript.

Reference Management Software: Use of EndNote is recommended for easy management and formatting of citations and reference lists.

Digital Object Identifier (DOI)

S. Karger Publishers supports DOIs as unique identifiers for articles. A DOI number will be printed on the title page of each article. DOIs can be useful in the future for identifying and citing articles published online without volume or issue information. More information can be found at www.doi.org.

Author's Choice™

Karger's Author's Choice service broadens the reach of your article and gives all users worldwide free and full access for reading, downloading and printing at www.karger.com. The option is available for a one-time fee of CHF 2750.–, which is a permissible cost in grant allocation. More information can be found at www.karger.com/authors_choice.

NIH-Funded Research

The U.S. National Institutes of Health (NIH) mandates under the NIH Public Access Policy that final, peer-reviewed manuscripts appear in its digital database within 12 months of the official publication date. As a service to authors, Karger submits the final version of your article on your behalf to PubMed Central. For those selecting our premium Author's Choice service, we will send your article immediately upon publishing, accelerating the accessibility of your work without the usual embargo. More details on NIH's Public Access Policy is available at http://publicaccess.nih.gov/FAQ.htm#a1

Self-Archiving

Karger permits authors to archive their pre-prints (i.e. prerefereeing) or post-prints (i.e. final draft post-refereeing) on their personal or institution's servers, provided the following conditions are met: Articles may not be used for commercial purposes, must be linked to the publisher's version, and must acknowledge the publisher's copyright. Authors selecting Karger's Author's Choice feature, however, are also permitted to archive the final, published version of their article, which includes copyediting and design improvements as well as citation links.

Proofs

Unless indicated otherwise, proofs are sent to the first-named author and should be returned with the least possible delay. Alterations made in proofs, other than the correction of printer's errors, are charged to the author. No page proofs are supplied.

Reprints

Order forms and a price list are sent with the proofs. Orders submitted after the issue is printed are subject to considerably higher prices.

KARGER

Fax +41 61 306 12 34
E-Mail karger@karger.ch
www.karger.com

The Guidelines for Authors are available at:
www.karger.com/nim_Guidelines

General Information

ISSN Print Edition: 1021–7401
ISSN Online Edition: 1423–0216

Journal Homepage: www.karger.com/nim

Publication Data: 'Neuroimmunomodulation' is published 6 times a year. Volume 17 with 6 issues appears in 2010.

Subscription Rates: Subscriptions run for a full calendar year. Prices are given per year.

Personal subscription:

Print or Online	Print+Online combined
CHF 578.90	CHF 623.90
EUR 413.35	EUR 445.35
USD 525.00	USD 568.00

postage and handling (added to print and print+online)
CHF 37.80 Europe, CHF 56.70 Overseas
EUR 27.–
USD 53.70

Institutional subscription:

Print or Online	Print+Online combined
CHF 1654.–	CHF 1819.–
EUR 1181.–	EUR 1299.–
USD 1500.00	USD 1650.00

postage and handling (added to print and print+online)
CHF 47.40 Europe, CHF 70.80 Overseas
EUR 33.60
USD 67.20

Airmail surcharge: CHF 48.– / USD 45.60

Please enquire about reduced rates for members of the: International Society of Neuroimmunomodulation

Back Volumes and Single Issues: Information on availability and prices of single print issues and print or electronic back volumes can be obtained from Customer Service at *service@karger.ch*.

Bibliographic Indices: This journal is regularly listed in bibliographic services, including *Current Contents®* and PubMed/MEDLINE.

Subscription Orders:
Orders can be placed at agencies, bookstores, directly with the Publisher

S. Karger AG
Medical and Scientific Publishers
P.O. Box
CH–4009 Basel
Switzerland
(for courier services only:
Allschwilerstrasse 10
CH–4055 Basel)
Tel. +41 61 306 11 11
Fax +41 61 306 12 34
E-Mail karger@karger.ch
www.karger.com

or further Karger offices or representatives:

France:
Librairie Medi-Sciences Sarl
36, bd de Latour-Maubourg
75007 Paris
France
Tél. +33 1 45 51 42 58
Fax +33 1 45 56 07 80
E-Mail librairie@medi-sciences.fr
www.medi-sciences.fr

Germany:
S. Karger GmbH
Postfach
79095 Freiburg
Deutschland
(Hausadresse: Wilhelmstrasse 20 A
79098 Freiburg)
Tel. +49 761 45 20 70
Fax +49 761 45 20 714
E-Post information@karger.de
www.karger.de

India, Bangladesh, Sri Lanka:
Panther Publishers Private Ltd.
33, First Main
Koramangala First Block
Bangalore 560 034
India
Tel. +91 80 25505 836
Tel. +91 80 25505 837
Fax +91 80 25505 981
E-Mail panther_publishers@vsnl.com
www.pantherpublishers.com

Japan:
Karger Japan, Inc.
Yushima S Bld. 3F
4-2-3, Yushima, Bunkyo-ku
Tokyo 113-0034
Japan
Tel. +81 3 3815 1800
Fax +81 3 3815 1802
E-Mail publisher@karger.jp

China, Taiwan and Malaysia:
Karger China
Suite 409, Apollo Building
1440 Central Yan An Road
Shanghai 200040
China
Tel. +86 21 6133 1861
Fax +86 21 6133 1862
E-Mail karger.ray@gmail.com

South America and Central America:
Cranbury International LLC
7 Clarendon Ave., Suite 2
Montpelier, VT 05602
USA
Tel. +1 802 223 6565
Fax +1 802 223 6824
E-Mail
eatkin@cranburyinternational.com
www.cranburyinternational.com

United Kingdom, Ireland:
S. Karger AG
c/o London Liaison Office
4 Rickett Street
London SW6 1RU
United Kingdom
Tel. +44 20 7386 0500
Fax +44 20 7610 3337
E-Mail uk@karger.ch

USA:
S. Karger Publishers, Inc.
26 West Avon Road
P.O. Box 529
Unionville, CT 06085
USA
Toll free: +1 800 828 5479
Tel. +1 860 675 7834
Fax +1 860 675 7302
E-Mail karger@snet.net

Change of Address:
Both old and new address should be sent to the subscription source.

KARGER

Fax +41 61 306 12 34
E-Mail karger@karger.ch
www.karger.com

The Journal Home Page is available at:
www.karger.com/nim

Proceedings of the 3rd Iberoamerican Congress on Neuroimmunomodulation

Buenos Aires, Argentina, 20–22 April, 2009

Editors
Claudia Pérez Leirós, Buenos Aires
Eduardo Arzt, Buenos Aires
Flavia Saravia, Buenos Aires
Valeria Rettori, Buenos Aires

18 figures, 1 in color, and 3 tables, 2010

KARGER Basel · Freiburg · Paris · London · New York · Bangalore · Bangkok · Shanghai · Singapore · Tokyo · Sydney

S. Karger
Medical and Scientific Publishers
Basel • Freiburg • Paris • London •
New York • Bangalore • Bangkok •
Shanghai • Singapore • Tokyo • Sydney

Disclaimer
The statements, opinions and data contained in this publication are solely those of the individual authors and contributors and not of the publisher and the editor(s). The appearance of advertisements in the journal is not a warranty, endorsement, or approval of the products or services advertised or of their effectiveness, quality or safety. The publisher and the editor(s) disclaim responsibility for any injury to persons or property resulting from any ideas, methods, instructions or products referred to in the content or advertisements.

Drug Dosage
The authors and the publisher have exerted every effort to ensure that drug selection and dosage set forth in this text are in accord with current recommendations and practice at the time of publication. However, in view of ongoing research, changes in government regulations, and the constant flow of information relating to drug therapy and drug reactions, the reader is urged to check the package insert for each drug for any change in indications and dosage and for added warnings and precautions. This is particularly important when the recommended agent is a new and/or infrequently employed drug.

Printed in Switzerland
on acid-free and non-aging paper (ISO 9706) by
Reinhardt Druck, Basel
ISBN 978–3–8055–9332–8
e-ISBN 978–3–8055–9333–5

KARGER

Fax +41 61 306 12 34
E-Mail karger@karger.ch
www.karger.com

NeuroImmunoModulation

Neuroimmunomodulation 2010;17:137–138
DOI: 10.1159/000258706

Published online: February 4, 2010

Preface

Claudia Pérez Leirós[a] Eduardo Arzt[b] Flavia Saravia[c] Valeria Rettori[d]

[a]Departamento de Química Biológica, Facultad de Ciencias Exactas y Naturales, y [b]Laboratorio de Fisiología y Biología Molecular y Celular, FCEN, Universidad de Buenos Aires, CONICET, [c]Instituto de Biología y Medicina Experimental, Facultad de Medicina, y [d]Centro de Estudios Farmacológicos y Botánicos, Facultad de Medicina, Universidad de Buenos Aires, Buenos Aires, Argentina

Buenos Aires was the venue of the Third Iberoamerican Congress of Neuroimmunomodulation, April 20–22, 2009, and the present compilation aims to update NIM readers with regard to the hot issues tackled by the speakers during the 3-day conferences.

As a compact overview of the whole program of the Congress, this special issue focuses on immunoneuroendocrine modulation from the standpoint of studying the mechanisms for the maintenance of homeostasis and the putative links between the loss of homeostatic control and the development of several disease states. The contributions were organized accordingly, with a first group of minireviews dealing with neuroimmune regulation in healthy conditions, and the next set of contributions discussing immunopathology, stress, neurodegeneration and aging.

Five minireviews concerning homeostasis open the proceedings, starting with Hugo Besedovsky's contribution that provides evidence of the homeostatic control of glucose by IL-1 and the modulation of synaptic plasticity by IL-1 and IL-6 which in turn influence learning and memory consolidation. This paper is followed by Wilson Savino's overview on the multivectorial process of T cell migration within the thymus that involves CXCL12 and semaphorin-3A among other molecules subject to neuroendocrine regulation. Susana Gonzalez then analyses the neuroprotective and promyelinating effects of progesterone in both the peripheral and central nervous system, including effects on the injured spinal cord; this section is completed by the reports on the endocannabinoid system as a modulator of early pregnancy and septic abortion described by Ana Franchi and of oxytocin and vasopressin production and secretion presented by Andrea De Laurentiis.

The next two contributions link the homeostatic control of the immune response by lectins and neuropeptides and its loss in inflammatory and autoimmune diseases with a review referring to galectins by Gabriel Rabinovich and that of vasoactive intestinal peptide and pituitary adenylyl cyclase activating peptide by Elena Gonzalez Rey.

The notion that neuroendocrine dysregulation underlies autoimmune, rheumatic and infectious diseases is then approached by Adriana del Rey's minireview on a collagen-induced model of rheumatoid arthritis; Jane Welsh's paper on the effects of stress on susceptibility to Theiler's virus-induced demyelination, a mouse model of multiple sclerosis; Marcelo Perone's report on the non-obese diabetic mouse model, and Maria Robinson's review on patients with neuromyelitis optica, an uncommon demyelinating disease. This set is completed with Waldemar Kanczkowski's report on Toll-like receptor

KARGER

Fax +41 61 306 12 34
E-Mail karger@karger.ch
www.karger.com

1021–7401/10/0173–0137$26.00/0

Accessible online at:
www.karger.com/nim

expression in human adrenocortical cells treated with bacterial-derived factors; Oscar Bottassos's overview of immunoendocrine disturbances on energy expenditure and the consumption state in tuberculosis patients, and Silvia Correa's work exploring the effects of stress on the spreading of fungal infection.

The final group of reviews deals with neuroimmune inputs in cognitive disorders, stress, neurodegeneration and ageing and starts with Moises Bauer's contribution on the immune impairment associated with post-traumatic stress disorders that develop following childhood abuse, and Joao Palermo Neto's overview of data generated over the past decade revealing that the effects of stressors on immunity and behavior highly depend on the experimental model as well as the frequency, duration, intensity, perception and the coping strategies of the stressed animal. This part continues with Andrea Marques' work exploring the biomarkers of stress in sweat (by cutaneous patches), heart rate and salivary cortisol in association with work environment in healthy subjects, and the review by Marta Romano on assessing the effects of acute and chronic stress by measuring glucocorticoids using noninvasive techniques in wild animals kept in the Zoo such as dolphins, and in wild felids and spider monkeys exposed to environmental changes. These papers are followed by Fernando Pitossi's work on the impairment of adult neurogenesis after prenatal LPS challenge in rats and Ricardo Maccioni's proposal of a neuroimmunomodulation theory of Alzheimer's disease based on the role of microglial activation that results in phosphorylation and self-aggregation of tau into neurotoxic oligomeric species. Finally, to close this special issue, the neuroendocrine regulation of immunity during aging is the focus of Monica de la Fuente's paper, evaluating immunosenescence and cognitive impairment as assessed by behavioral tests in prematurely aged animals, and Agustin Zapata's report on the CXCL12/CXCR4 ligand/receptor pair as a physiological regulator of homeostasis in the human thymus during aging.

To end this preface, we would like to thank all the speakers for sending their short reviews in a timely manner so that this special issue of *Neuroimmunomodulation* could be promptly realized.

NeuroImmunoModulation

Neuroimmunomodulation 2010;17:139–141
DOI: 10.1159/000258707

Published online: February 4, 2010

Interleukin-1 Resets Glucose Homeostasis at Central and Peripheral Levels: Relevance for Immunoregulation

Hugo O. Besedovsky Adriana del Rey

Department of Immunophysiology, Institute of Physiology and Pathophysiology, Medical Faculty, Marburg, Germany

Key Words
Interleukin-1 · Glucose homeostasis · Immunoregulation · Immune-brain interactions

Abstract
We briefly discuss here evidence showing that the capacity of IL-1β to mediate adjustments of glucose homeostasis can be added to the already well-known pleiotropic effects of this cytokine. Such adjustments, which are necessary for satisfying the high energetic demands of immune/inflammatory responses, can be mediated by effects of endogenous IL-1 exerted at peripheral and brain levels in a concerted action with other cytokines and neuroendocrine mechanisms.

Glucose is the main fuel for immune cells and the immune response is a process which is highly demanding in terms of energy [1]. Glucose uptake markedly increases in activated immune cells, in which its transport is predominantly mediated by GLUT1 [1–3] indicating a deviation of glucose supply towards the immune system. This effect is facilitated by the capacity of IL-1 and TNF-α to induce insulin resistance [3], and will preferentially affect tissues such as skeletal muscle and fat in which glucose uptake is mainly mediated by the insulin-dependent transporter GLUT4. Thus, because of a defective insulin control, glucose homeostasis is considerably altered during diseases that involve the immune system [3]. However, to certain extent, alteration of glucose homeostasis is a necessary price to pay for 'feeding' immune cells.

Although in the following we shall refer to the role of IL-1 in providing energy support to the immune system, it should not to be forgotten that this cytokine is usually released together with other mediators that can have opposite actions.

Role of IL-1 in Glucoregulation

While most hormones and the catecholamines increase glucose blood levels, insulin is considered to have the 'monopoly' in inducing hypoglycemia. However, we have shown that exogenous and endogenous IL-1 can induce a prolonged hypoglycemia, a surprising effect due to the capacity of the cytokine to increase glucocorticoid levels [4]. The hypoglycemic effect is not mediated by insulin since it is also observed in insulin-resistant, type 2 diabetic animals, and is dissociable from pyrogenic, anorexic, and inflammatory effects of the cytokine [4–6]. The dissociation of hypoglycemic from deleterious inflammatory effects of IL-1 is important because it has

KARGER

Fax +41 61 306 12 34
E-Mail karger@karger.ch
www.karger.com

1021–7401/10/0173–0139$26.00/0

Accessible online at:
www.karger.com/nim

Prof. Dr. Hugo O. Besedovsky
Department of Immunophysiology, Institute of Physiology and Pathophysiology
Medical Faculty, Deutschhausstrasse 2, DE–35037 Marburg (Germany)
Tel. +49 6421 286 2174, Fax +49 6421 286 8925
E-Mail besedovs@mailer.uni-marburg.de

been shown that this cytokine is involved in the pathogenesis of type 1 diabetes by affecting pancreatic β-cells [see references in 7].

At peripheral levels, the effect of IL-1 is mediated by increased glucose transport in GLUT1- and GLUT3-expressing tissues, including immune cells [1]. IL-1-induced hypoglycemia is long-lasting and far more prolonged than that of regular insulin. For example, intraperitoneal injection of nanogram amounts of the cytokine into mice results in about 50% reduction in glucose blood levels, the effect is still not completely extinguished after 18–24 h. IL-1 induces hepatic glycogen depletion and inhibits gluconeogenesis [6, 8, for further references, see 9]. In parallel to hypoglycemia, IL-1 induces an early counter-regulatory response, involving increased glucagon, catecholamine and glucocorticoids secretion, but these changes are surprisingly short-lasting and disappear after 4 h, about the time of maximal reduction in glucose blood levels induced by IL-1. In normal rats, IL-1-induced hypoglycemia is less marked, but it is paralleled by a clear compensatory decrease in insulin secretion [6]. An initial hyperglycemia that can be followed by hypoglycemia is noticed in septic patients, in which different cytokines are overproduced, and there is an important increase in glucose expenditure that is not mediated by insulin [for review, see 3].

IL-1 Provides Energy to Support Immune Responses

While IL-3 and IL-7 contribute to provide energy for hematopoiesis and to quiescent immune cells, respectively [1], there is evidence that IL-1 can supply fuel support during immune responses, since it can induce glucose uptake in different tissues, including lymphoid organs [8]. Besides its pro-inflammatory and adjuvant actions and its capacity to activate a cytokine network, IL-1 acts as a costimulatory signal for T cells, either directly or through interactions with other co-stimulatory molecules, such as B7/CD28, and is an inducer of IL-2 and IL-17 [7]. Its capacity to induce glucose uptake suggests that IL-1 is a major candidate to supply glucose to immune cells for essential processes such as phagocytosis, proliferation, clonal expansion, and generation of effector mediators and cells. Although insulin is an important growth factor for immune cells, the effect of IL-1 is largely independent of that of insulin. As mentioned, both molecules act via different glucose transporters, and the hypoglycemic effect of IL-1 is even more profound in insulin-resistant diabetic animals [5].

Evidence that IL-1 Can Change the Set Point of Glucoregulation at Brain Levels

Due to the strict control of glycemia, which under health conditions depends on the balance between insulin and counterregulatory neuroendocrine mechanisms, a redistribution of glucose supply during disease to favor the activity of immune cells cannot be sustained without a change in the set point of glucoregulation. We have recently shown that IL-1, produced and acting in the brain, changes this set point during activation of peripheral immune cells [9]. Hypoglycemia normally induces an increase in food intake, a response that is controlled by glucoregulatory centers in the brain. The long-lasting hypoglycemic effect of IL-1, the inhibition of a counterregulatory feedback, and the lack of a compensatory increase in food intake suggest that the cytokine induces a change in the set point of glucoregulation. This change in the set point is also manifested by the fact that normal and type II diabetic animals treated with IL-1 and challenged with a glucose load not only show an accelerated glucose clearance (probably due to a peripheral component) but return to the hypoglycemic values attained by injection of the cytokine [4, 5]. Direct evidence that IL-1 changes the set point of glucoregulation by acting at brain levels is based on results showing that: (a) central administration of IL-1β reduces glucose levels; (b) blockade of IL-1 receptors in the brain mediates a quick return to euglycemia after a glucose load in IL-1β-treated, normal and diabetic mice; (c) IL-1β gene expression is markedly increased in the hypothalamus of normal and diabetic mice treated with IL-1β or LPS, and (d) IL-1β mRNA transcripts in the hypothalamus negatively correlate with glucose blood levels in normal and diabetic mice treated with IL-1β [9 and further references in this publication].

Conclusion: Immunoregulatory Relevance of Central and Peripheral Effects of IL-1 on Glucose Homeostasis

Interestingly, the concept of homeostasis, a term coined by W. Cannon, derives from the discovery by C. Bernard that, although the concentration of sugar in blood can be raised or lowered by a number of processes, the net outcome of these processes is to keep blood sugar concentration within certain limits. Today, it is known that several neuroendocrine regulatory mechanisms integrated at brain levels contribute to maintain this constancy around a preset value. However, homeostasis needs to be adaptive, since it is necessary to adjust set points and reprogramme regulatory mechanisms when circumstances require. Probably the most obvious situation is the transition from health to disease and, if the course is successful for the organism, the return to health. Under health conditions, the priority is to provide glucose mainly to skeletal muscle and brain, and to prepare the host for an eventual acute stress (flight or fight response). During diseases that imply a strong activation of the immune system, such as infections, the priority is to provide energy, predominately derived from glycolysis, to support immune cell activity. Indeed, the immune system is probably the only bodily system that requires cell proliferation and clonal expansion to fulfill its physiologic functions. The energy required, mainly due to immune cell proliferation, is illustrated by the fact that during infective, inflammatory, and autoimmune diseases, secondary lymphoid organs abruptly grow (lymph node enlargement, splenomegaly), reaching a several-fold bigger mass than in healthy individuals. Such increase can be noticed already hours or few days after infection. Because of the effects described above, IL-1 can be positioned centrally in mediating a resetting of glucose homeostasis. The cytokine can be released locally in lymphoid organs and at infective/inflammatory foci, stimulate glucose uptake and glycolytic processes in immune cells, and cause insulin resistance in other tissues. During disease, peripheral and brain-borne IL-1 conveys signals to the hypothalamus, where glucose-sensing neurons are located. A re-programming of glucoregulatory mechanisms is necessary to favor immune processes, because the brain also receives other, non-immunologic signals that tend to keep the 'status quo'. Nevertheless, the final result is that counterregulatory responses are inhibited by brain-borne IL-1. In mice, this effect results in a marked hypoglycemia. However, locally released IL-1, acting in an autocrine/paracrine way, would favor glucose supply to immune cells at the expense of insulin-sensitive tissues, with a restricted cost for the brain. In other species, for example the rat, the local effect of IL-1 on pancreatic β-cells [7], and the brain-mediated reduction of insulin output combined with resistance to the hormone can also favour a preferential redistribution of glucose supply during immune processes.

Taken together, the effect of IL-1 on glucose homeostasis constitutes a further evidence of the relevance of interactions between the immune, nervous, and endocrine systems for immunoregulation. As with other physiologic mechanisms, a deregulation of IL-1 production or action can contribute to disease. For example, long-lasting IL-1 overproduction in normal mice results in hypoglycemia, increased glucose utilization, and a lean phenotype [8], while the absence of IL-1 signals in IL-1 receptor type I knockout or in transgenic mice overexpressing IL-1 receptor antagonist induces type 2 diabetes [11, 12]. However, in genetically predisposed individuals, the local inflammatory effect of IL-1 on pancreatic β-cells can contribute to the pathogenesis of diabetes type 1 [references in 7].

Acknowledgement

This work was supported by the German Research Council (DFG; RE 1451/3-1).

References

1 Fox CJ, Hammerman PS, Thompson CB: Fuel feeds function: energy metabolism and the T-cell response. Nat Rev Immunol 2005;5:844–852.
2 Fukuzumi M, Shinomiya H, Shimizu Y, Ohishi K, Utsumi S: Endotoxin-induced enhancement of glucose influx into murine peritoneal macrophages via GLUT1. Infect Immun 1996;64:108–112.
3 McGuinness OP: Defective glucose homeostasis during infection. Annu Rev Nutr 2005;25:9–35.
4 del Rey A, Besedovsky H: Interleukin 1 affects glucose homeostasis. Am J Physiol 1987;253:R794–R798.
5 del Rey A, Besedovsky H: Antidiabetic effects of interleukin 1. Proc Natl Acad Sci USA 1989;86:5943–5947.
6 Besedovsky HO, del Rey A: Immune-neuro-endocrine interactions: facts and hypotheses. Endocr Rev 1996;17:64–102.
7 Dinarello CA: Immunological and inflammatory functions of the interleukin-1 family. Annu Rev Immunol 2009;27:519–550.
8 Metzger S, Nusair S, Planer D, Barash V, Pappo O, Shilyansky J, Chajek-Shaul T: Inhibition of hepatic gluconeogenesis and enhanced glucose uptake contribute to the development of hypoglycemia in mice bearing interleukin-1beta-secreting tumor. Endocrinology 2004;145:5150–5156.
9 del Rey A, Roggero E, Randolf A, Mahuad C, McCann S, Rettori V, Besedovsky HO: IL-1 resets glucose homeostasis at central levels. Proc Natl Acad Sci USA 2006;103:16039–16044.
10 Ota K, Wildmann J, Ota T, Besedovsky HO, del Rey A: Interleukin-1beta and insulin elicit different neuroendocrine responses to hypoglycemia. Ann NY Acad Sci 2009;1153:82–88.
11 Matsuki T, Horai R, Sudo K, Iwakura Y: IL-1 plays an important role in lipid metabolism by regulating insulin levels under physiological conditions. J Exp Med 2003;198:877–888.
12 Garcia MC, Wernstedt I, Berndtsson A, Enge M, Bell M, Hultgren O, Horn M, Ahrén B, Enerback S, Ohlsson C, Wallenius V, Jansson JO: Mature-onset obesity in interleukin-1 receptor I knockout mice. Diabetes 2006;55:1205–1213.

NeuroImmunoModulation

Neuroimmunomodulation 2010;17:142–145
DOI: 10.1159/000258708

Published online: February 4, 2010

Intrathymic T Cell Migration Is a Multivectorial Process under a Complex Neuroendocrine Control

Wilson Savino

Laboratory on Thymus Research, Oswaldo Cruz Institute, Oswaldo Cruz Foundation, Rio de Janeiro, Brazil

Key Words

Thymocyte migration · Thymic microenvironment · Laminin · Fibronectin · Integrins · Chemokines · Semaphorins · Neuropilins

Abstract

The thymus is responsible for normal T cell development, a process that includes cell proliferation, death, migration, and T cell receptor gene rearrangements. Moreover, it depends on interactions between developing thymocytes and thymic microenvironmental cells. Along with differentiation, thymocytes migrate and such oriented movement is regulated by several molecular interactions, comprising extracellular matrix (ECM) elements and chemokines. We postulated that intrathymic T cell migration is a multivectorial process; each individual vector being represented by a given molecular interaction. In vivo and in vitro experiments revealed that migration of developing thymocytes, including the export of mature T cells, is upregulated by hormones, such as growth hormone and triiodothyronine, through the modulation of ECM-mediated interactions, associated or not with the chemokine CXCL12. Recent data revealed that molecular interactions typically found in the nervous system also affect intrathymic T cell migration. Semaphorin-3A, a soluble member of the semaphorin family, is involved in the control of human thymocyte migration, bearing a chemorepulsive role. Such an effect is partially due to its downregulatory effect upon the interactions mediated by fibronectin and laminin, as well as CXCL12. These data unravel a complex neuroendocrine control intrathymic T cell migration, involving both endocrine and paracrine molecular interactions.

The thymus is the primary lymphoid organ, where bone-marrow-derived T cell precursors differentiate, ultimately leading to migration of positively selected thymocytes to the peripheral lymphoid organs where they will specifically find *niches* in the T cell-dependent areas. This process involves expression of various proteins and rearrangements of T cell receptor (TCR) genes. Most immature thymocytes do not express TCR, CD4 or CD8 molecules, being called double-negative ($CD4^-CD8^-$) cells, representing 5% of thymic lymphocytes. As they progress in maturation, they acquire CD4 and CD8 markers, generating the $CD4^+CD8^+$ cells, comprising 80% of the whole population. At this stage, TCR genes are completely rearranged. Thymocytes that do not undergo productive TCR gene rearrangement die by apoptosis, whereas those expressing productive TCR will interact with peptides presented by the major histocompatibility com-

KARGER

Fax +41 61 306 12 34
E-Mail karger@karger.ch
www.karger.com

1021–7401/10/0173–0142$26.00/0

Accessible online at:
www.karger.com/nim

Wilson Savino
Laboratory on Thymus Research, Oswaldo Cruz Institute, Oswaldo Cruz Foundation
Ave. Brasil 4365, Manguinhos, Rio de Janeiro, RJ 21045-900 (Brazil)
Tel. +55 21 3865 8101, Fax +55 21 3865 8250
E-Mail savino@fiocruz.br, w_savino@hotmail.com

plex expressed by microenvironmental cells. This interaction determines positive and negative selection events: positively selected thymocytes progress to the mature $TCR^+CD4^+CD8^-$ or $TCR^+CD4^-CD8^+$ single-positive stage (comprising 15% of thymocytes), which can be exported to peripheral lymphoid organs [1].

The thymic microenvironment also influences thymocyte differentiation via cytokines, chemokines, adhesion molecules and extracellular matrix (ECM), most of which modulate not only differentiation but also thymocyte migration patterns [2, 3]. The thymic epithelial cell (TEC) network is the major component of the thymic microenvironment, being responsible for positive selection of thymocytes, and for the production of cytokines, chemokines and various ECM components [3]. It is a heterogeneous tissue, and TEC in different locations within the thymic lobules may be related to specific steps in T cell maturation. One cortically located lymphoepithelial complex, which can be isolated ex vivo is the thymic nurse cell (TNC), being formed by one TEC that harbors large amounts of differentiating thymocytes. Once in culture, TNCs release thymocytes, and TNC-derived epithelial cells can reconstitute lymphoepithelial complexes after being co-cultured with immature thymocytes. These features places TNC as an in vitro model of thymocyte migration within the TEC context [3, 4].

Thymocyte differentiation occurs as cells migrate within the thymic lobules: immature $TCR^-CD4^-CD8^-$ and $TCR^+CD4^+CD8^+$ cells are cortically located, whereas mature $TCR^+CD4^+CD8^-$ and $TCR^+CD4^-CD8^+$ lymphocytes are found in the medulla. Such migration is complex, being controlled by several molecular interactions, including those mediated by ECM and chemokines [3].

It is now established that the thymus is under neuroendocrine control, with several hormones, neuropeptides and neurotransmitters being able to affect a variety of thymic functions [4].

Hormones Modulate the Entrance of T Cell Precursors into the Thymus

Although studies on the neuroendocrine control of the entrance of T cell precursors into the thymus are still scarce, it was reported that GH increases human T cell engraftment into the thymus of severe combined immunodeficiency syndrome mice; an effect mediated by β1 and β2 integrin receptors. This is in keeping with data showing that the entrance of bone marrow-derived progenitors into the organ is partly mediated by the VCAM-1/fibronectin receptor, the integrin α4β1 [reviewed in ref. 5].

Hormones Upregulate Thymocyte Migration via ECM-Mediated Interactions

Treatment of cultured TEC with GH or triiodothyronine (T_3) yielded an increase in the amounts of fibronectin and laminin, and in the expression of their corresponding receptors, VLA-5 and VLA-6 [4, 6]. Since thymocyte/TEC adhesion is partly mediated by ECM, we tested whether these hormones were able to modulate this interaction. In fact, thymocyte adhesion to cultured TEC is enhanced by GH and T_3. This effect could be prevented in TEC cultures pretreated with anti-ECM or anti-ECM receptor antibodies [4–6]. Together, these data indicate that ECM-mediated TEC/thymocyte adhesion, which is crucial for intrathymic T cell traffic, is under hormonal control. Accordingly, thymocyte traffic in the context of TNC, which is also mediated by ECM [3], is enhanced by GH and T_3, with a significantly acceleration of thymocyte release from TNCs and increase in the entrance of thymocytes to reconstitute new lymphoepithelial complexes [4–6]. We also noticed that the production of laminin by TNCs derived from GH-transgenic mice is increased compared to wild-type control mice and that thymocyte release from TNCs was also faster in GH-transgenic animals [6].

Growth Hormone Stimulates Thymocyte Migration by a Combined Effect of Laminin and CXCL12

The effects of GH upon thymocyte migration were also approached ex vivo by using transwell migration chambers. We observed an enhanced laminin-driven thymocyte migration in GH-transgenic mice, when compared with wild-type animals, although the expression of the laminin receptor VLA-6 on thymocytes from GH-transgenic mice did not change significantly. This implies that the activation of this integrin is higher when GH contents are increased. Since intrathymic laminin deposition is also enhanced in vivo in these animals, it is likely that hyperresponsive thymocytes, encountering higher amounts of laminin, accelerate their traffic within the organ.

GH also modulates other interactions related to thymocyte migration: CXCL12-driven migration is higher

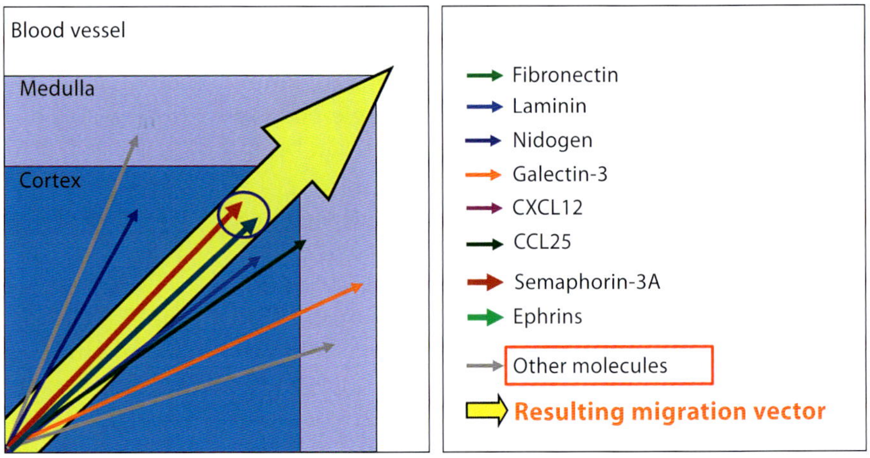

Fig. 1. Concept of multivectorial thymocyte migration, including semaphorin-3A and ephrins as novel cell migration vectors. The panel schematically defines the hypothetical concept stating that the thymocyte migration results from a balance of several simultaneous ligand/receptor pair interactions [15]. Accordingly, individual vectors form a resulting vector that leads thymocytes throughout their journey within the thymic lobules, from the cortex toward the medulla, with mature subsets ultimately being exported from the organ through the blood vessel walls. Accordingly, those vectors that are under neuroendocrine control, once modulated by a given hormone or neuropeptide, will likely alter the resulting vector. Narrow arrows represent individual migration vectors induced by specific stimuli including ECM ligands such as fibronectin, laminin, nidogen and galectin-3, chemokines such as CXCL12 and CCL25, semaphorin-3A, ephrins and other yet to be defined molecules. Dashed arrows represent the final resulting migration vector.

in GH-transgenic mice compared with control animals, although the membrane levels of CXCR4 remained unchanged in both transgenic and wild-type animals, suggesting that CXCR4 is also spontaneously activated in GH-transgenic thymocytes [5, 6]. Conjointly, these data indicate that the enhanced thymocyte migration seen in GH-transgenic and in GH-injected mice results at least partly from a combined action of laminin and CXCL12.

Hormones Can Modulate Thymocyte Export

One in vivo strategy to evaluate thymocyte export is the evaluation of recent thymic emigrants (RTEs). It is well established that intrathymic injection of fluorescein isothiocyanate (FITC) labels thymocytes, allowing the recovery of the FITC$^+$ cells that have recently been exported. Following intrathymic injection of normal mice with GH in combination with FITC, we found a significant increase in the percentages of CD4$^+$CD8$^-$FITC$^+$ cells in the lymph nodes; the same being observed when FITC was injected within the thymus of GH-transgenic animals [5, 7].

These data are in keeping with previous reports showing an increase in human RTEs in the blood of AIDS patients who received GH in conjunction with specific antiretrovirus therapy [8]. Interestingly, AIDS patients develop severe thymic atrophy and a decrease in GH levels [5]. Accordingly, long-term GH treatment augmented thymus volume concomitantly with an enhanced export of CD4$^+$ T cells [8]. Of note, animals treated with T_3 also export more RTEs to lymph nodes [9].

Intrathymic Molecular Interactions Typically Found in the Nervous System

In addition to the circuitry discussed above, several molecules involved in the crosstalk between neural cells during brain development are expressed in the thymus. For example, ephrins and their receptors Ephs are highly expressed in the nervous system during development and were described as important in growth cone collapse and cell detachment [10]. Recently, the expression of ephrins and Ephs has been reported in thymocytes and thymic microenvironmental cells. EphA4, B2 and B3 knockout mice present altered thymocyte development suggesting that these molecules could be important in the organization of the thymus and thymocyte migration. In this respect, it was shown that some Eph ligands as ephrins A1, A3 and B2 can inhibit the CXCL12-induced chemotaxis of human thymocytes [11].

In a second vein, the cellular prion protein (PrP^C), mainly expressed in nervous tissues, is also expressed in the thymus. Interestingly, mouse overexpressing PrP^C present thymic hypoplasia with accumulation of CD4-CD8 double-negative cells [12]. We showed that in addition to the hypoplasia of the organ, thymocytes from PrP^C transgenic mice do not respond to laminin in terms of cell migration [13], thus placing PrP^C as a further player in intrathymic T cell migration.

We also reported in the intrathymic expression of another ligand/receptor pair originally described in the nervous system: neuropilin-1 (NP-1) and its respective ligand semaphorin-3A. In the human thymus, NP1 is expressed in low percentages of thymocytes (although comprising all CD4/CD8-defined subsets) and at high levels by TECs and dendritic cells. Semaphorin-3A downregulates human thymocyte adhesion onto TEC monolayers, as pre-incubation of thymocytes with this molecule resulted in 50% inhibition of adhesion of all CD4/CD8-defined thymocyte subsets. Furthermore, semaphorin-3A exerts per se a chemorepulsive effect and also inhibits fibronectin and laminin-induced thymocyte migration, showing the importance of semaphorin-3A/NP-1 interactions in thymocyte guidance, alone or combined with other molecules as ECM ligands [14].

Concluding Remarks

The data discussed above reinforce the notion that thymocyte migration is complex, comprising multiple combined molecular interactions leading to chemoattraction or chemorepulsion, involving various molecules like ECM ligands, chemokines, ephrins and semaphorins in a concept proposed as multivectorial migration [15] (fig. 1). This resulting vector can be altered by hormones and/or neuropeptides able to modulate one or more cell migration-related molecular interactions within the organ. Actually, we preclude that further 'neuroimmune' interactions will be reported to be involved in intrathymic cell migration.

Overall, the data summarized herein unravel a complex neuroendocrine control intrathymic T cell migration, involving endocrine and paracrine molecular interactions. Lastly, we can take advantage of this knowledge to design therapeutic approaches in pathological situations, by targeting specific molecular interactions of this type of neuroendocrine control.

Acknowledgements

This work was funded with grants by Fiocruz, CNPq and CAPES (Brazil), being developed in the context of the CNRS-Fiocruz Associated Laboratory of Immunology and Immunopathology.

References

1 Ciofani M, Zúñiga-Pflücker JC: The thymus as an inductive site for T lymphopoiesis. Annu Rev Cell Dev Biol 2007;23:463–493.
2 Savino W, Mendes-da-Cruz DA, Smaniotto S, Silva-Monteiro E, Villa-Verde DMS: Control of thymocyte migration: an interplay of distinct cellular interactions. J Leukocyte Biol 2004;75:951–961.
3 Petrie HT, Zúñiga-Pflücker JC: Zoned out: functional mapping of stromal signaling microenvironments in the thymus. Annu Rev Immunol 2007;25:649–679.
4 Savino W, Dardenne M: Neuroendocrine control of thymus physiology. Endocrine Rev 2000;21:412–443.
5 Savino W: Neuroendocrine control of T cell development in mammals: role of growth hormone in modulating thymocyte migration. Exp Physiol 2007;92:813–817.
6 Ribeiro-Carvalho MM, Farias-de-Oliveira DA, Villa-Verde DMS, Savino W: Triiodothyronine modulates extracellular matrix-mediated interactions between thymocytes and thymic microenvironmental cells. Neuroimmunomodulation 2002;75:139–150.
7 Smaniotto S, Mello-Coelho V, Villa-Verde DMS, Pléau JM, Postel-Vinay MC, Dardenne M, Savino W: Growth hormone modulates thymocyte development in vivo through a combined action of laminin and CXCL12. Endocrinology 2005;146:3005–3017.
8 Napolitano LA, Schmidt D, Gotway MB, Ameli N, Filbert EL, Ng MM, Clor JL, Epling L, Sinclair E, Baum PD, Li K, Killian ML, Bacchetti P, McCune JM: Growth hormone enhances thymic function in HIV-1-infected adults. J Clin Invest 2008;118:1085–1098.
9 Ribeiro-Carvalho MM, Smaniotto S, Neves-dos-Santos S, Mouço T, Savino W, Mello-Coelho V: Triiodothyronine modulates differential homing of recent thymic emigrants to peripheral lymphoid organs. Scand J Immunol 2007;66:8–16.
10 Pasquale E: Eph-ephrin bidirectional signaling in physiology and disease. Cell 2008;133: 38–52.
11 Muñoz JJ, García-Ceca J, Alfaro D, Stimamiglio MA, Cejalvo T, Jiménez E, Zapata AG: Organizing the thymus gland. Ann NY Acad Sci 2009;1153:14–19.
12 Jouvin-Marche E, Attuil-Audenis V, Aude-Garcia C, Rachidi W, Zabel M, Podevin-Dimster V, Siret C, Huber C, Martinic M, Riondel J, Villiers CL, Favier A, Naquet P, Cesbron JY, Marche PN: Overexpression of cellular prion protein induces an antioxidant environment altering T cell development in the thymus. J Immunol 2006;176:3490–3497.
13 Terra-Granado E, Berbert LR, de Meis J, Nomizo R, Martins VR, Savino W, Silva-Barbosa SD: Is there a role for cellular prion protein in intrathymic T cell differentiation and migration? Neuroimmunomodulation 2007; 14:213–219.
14 Lepelletier Y, Smaniotto S, Hadj-Slimane R, Villa-Verde DMS, Nogueira AC, Dardenne M, Hermine H, Savino W: Control of human thymocyte migration by neuropilin-1/semaphorin-3A-mediated interactions. Proc Natl Acad Sci USA 2007;104:5545–5550.
15 Mendes-da-Cruz DA, Smaniotto S, Keller AC, Dardenne M, Savino W: Multivectorial abnormal cell migration in the NOD mouse thymus. J Immunol 2008;180:4639–4647.

NeuroImmunoModulation

Neuroimmunomodulation 2010;17:146–149
DOI: 10.1159/000258709

Published online: February 4, 2010

Progesterone and the Spinal Cord: Good Friends in Bad Times

Florencia Labombarda María Claudia González Deniselle
Alejandro Federico De Nicola Susana Laura González

Laboratorio de Bioquímica Neuroendócrina, Instituto de Biología y Medicina Experimental, CONICET, Obligado 2490, C1428ADN, Buenos Aires, Argentina

Key Words
Spinal cord injury · Progesterone · Brain-derived neurotrophic factor · Oligodendrocytes · Remyelination

Abstract
In recent years, a growing list of publications point to the value of steroid hormones as an interesting option for the treatment of several type of lesions and diseases of the nervous system. Progesterone, well known for its role in pregnancy, has recently been shown to exert neuroprotective and promyelinating effects in both, the peripheral and central nervous system, including the injured spinal cord. Previous work from our laboratory has shown that progesterone actions in experimental models of spinal neurodegeneration or injury may involve the modulation of brain-derived neurotrophic factor, a neurotrophin with important implications in neuronal survival and axonal regeneration. The spinal cord is target for progesterone since neurons and glial cells express the intracellular receptors for this neuroactive steroid. However, the presence in the spinal cord of new membrane receptors and the enzymes involved in progesterone metabolism to its reduced derivatives, which modulate the activity of neurotransmitter receptors, suggest that progesterone actions involve pleiotropic mechanisms. Our recent data uncovering several molecular events may help to understand the protective and promyelinating actions of progesterone and further support the role of this steroid as a promising therapeutic agent for neurotrauma and/or neurodegenerative diseases.

Spinal cord injury (SCI) is a devastating condition that affects all cell types populating the spinal cord and causes marked pathological changes, including early motoneuron degeneration, activation of astroglial and microglial cells and secondary demyelination [1, 2]. The neuronal response to spinal injury includes several landmarks of cell damage, as the development of nuclear eccentricity and dissolution of Nissl bodies (chromatolytic changes), the loss of microtubule-associated proteins and a decreased expression of several key enzymes for the normal neuronal function [2–5].

In addition, mature oligodendrocytes, the source of myelin proteins in the central nervous system, are extremely sensitive to the effects of injury [6]. After spinal trauma, several factors as glutamate excitotoxicity, oxidative stress and pro-inflammatory cytokines may contribute to the injury-induced oligodendrocyte death and secondary demyelination. Successful remyelination requires the proliferation of oligodendrocytes precursors cells (OPC), which express the proteoglycan NG2 surface marker, and their differentiation into myelin-producing

KARGER

Fax +41 61 306 12 34
E-Mail karger@karger.ch
www.karger.com

1021–7401/10/0173–0146$26.00/0

Accessible online at:
www.karger.com/nim

Susana Laura González, PhD
Facultad de Medicina, Universidad de Buenos Aires
Paraguay 2155, Buenos Aires C1121ABG (Argentina)
Tel. +54 11 4783 2869, Fax +54 11 4786 2564
E-Mail sugonza@dna.uba.ar

oligodendrocytes, that can be labeled as $CC1^+$ cells. The oligodendrocyte linage undergoes a complex process from OPC to mature oligodendrocytes and involves the participation of several transcription factors (Olig1, Olig2 and Nkx2.2) with specific roles during OPC differentiation and remyelination. However, this process is incomplete after SCI. For this reason, the search of agents that stimulate and/or protect the cellular regeneration programs represents a challenging area of neurobiological research.

In recent years, progesterone (PROG), a steroid classically associated with reproductive functions, has been shown to exert neuroprotective, promyelinating and anti-inflammatory effects in both the peripheral and central nervous system [6]. These observations have stimulated further research to uncover the effectiveness of PROG to treat traumatic, neurodegenerative or autoimmune disease [6].

In this report we summarize our recent results exploring the effects of PROG as a novel neuroprotective and promyelinating agent for the injured spinal cord that may help to support its role as a therapeutic agent for the treatment of central trauma and disease.

Neuroprotective Effects of Progesterone after Spinal Cord Injury

Early work from our laboratory shows that the injured spinal cord is a target for the neuroprotective actions of PROG [3]. In spinal motoneurones, PROG upregulates some key proteins that are necessary for neuronal function both after trauma and in a mouse model of neurodegeneration [2, 3, 6]. In this regard, PROG restores both injured-decreased expression of the Na,K-ATPase subunits and the cholinergic marker choline acetyltransferase (ChAT), whereas it further increased the growth-associated protein GAP-43. These are considered important neuroprotective responses since ChAT catalyzes acetylcholine synthesis, which is responsible to start the muscle contraction at the neuromuscular junction. In addition, the sodium pump maintains the membrane potential, neuronal excitability and the entrance of ions and nutrients into the soma, whereas GAP-43 is involved in axonal regeneration. Further data regarding the neuroprotective effects of PROG were obtained exploring the notion that neurotrophins and steroid hormones are able to interplay in the central nervous system. In particular, our interest was focused on brain-derived neurotrophic factor (BDNF) since it mimics the effects of PROG on the mentioned parameters when administered to animals after axotomy or spinal trauma. Thus, to clarify whether endogenous BDNF expression could be regulated by PROG, we employed in situ hybridization as well as immunohistochemistry to analyze changes in BDNF mRNA and protein, respectively. In these studies, male Sprague-Dawley rats were sham-operated or underwent complete spinal cord transection at thoracic level. Animals received oil vehicle or four injections of PROG (4 mg/kg b.w.) at 1, 24, 48 and 72 h (s.c.) postinjury. In the injured animals, SCI causes a marked depletion of both BDNF mRNA and protein expression that is coincident with intense chromatolytic changes [4] and down-regulation of ChAT and Na,K-ATPase expression [3]. However, a 3-day course of PROG administration to the injured animals enhances 200% mRNA BDNF in ventral horn motoneurons and significantly upregulates protein expression as compared to untreated animals [4]. At this time period, PROG also prevents the lesion-induced chromatolytic changes [4] that were further confirmed at the ultrastructural level [5]. In addition, we also observed that PROG preserves the microtubule-associated protein 2 (MAP2) immunostaining in deafferentiated motoneurones, which may help to recover cytoskeleton organization [5]. Collectively, our results and those from a recent report [7] suggest that PROG-induced BDNF expression correlates with its neuroprotective effects and may help to understand the potential role of PROG to support and sustain normal cellular function after SCI.

Promyelinating Effects of Progesterone after Spinal Cord Injury

In addition to its role as a neuroprotective factor, PROG is also emerging as a promyelinating molecule in the nervous system. In a recent report [8], we have employed the complete spinal cord transection model to study whether PROG may influence OPC proliferation and their differentiation into myelinating oligodendrocytes.

To accomplish this goal, we administered vehicle or PROG (16 mg/kg/day) to the animals with spinal cord injury, which were euthanized 3 or 21 days postinjury. The phenotype of pure OPC cells was assessed using a double-labeling immunofluorescence protocol, in which cells were exposed to NG2 staining followed by anti-Ox42 antibody, to discard the contribution of microglia or macrophages to the $NG2^+$ population. Single-labeled cells ($NG2^+/Ox42^-$) were indicative of OPC and were

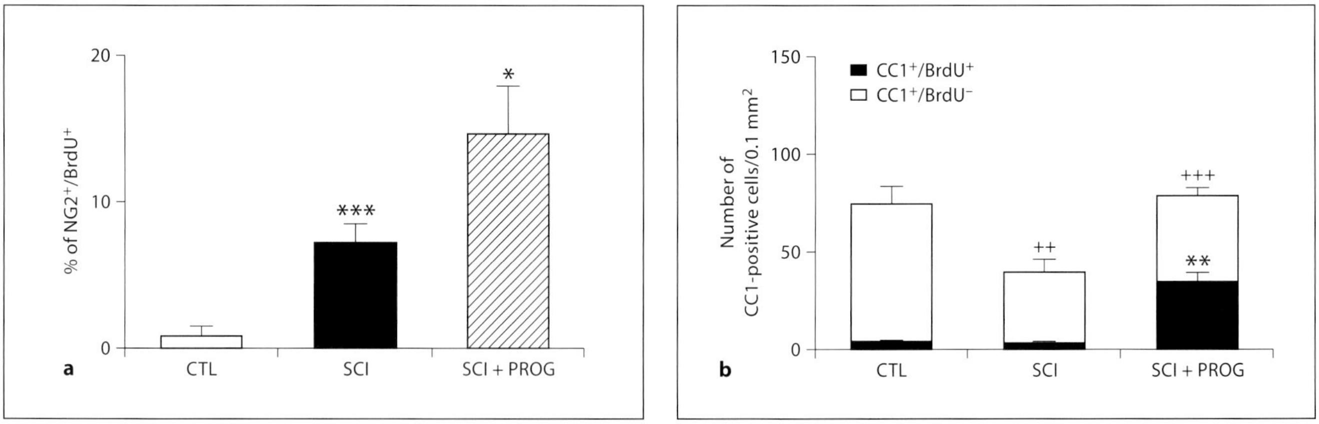

Fig. 1. a Effects of SCI and PROG administration on the proliferation of NG2 cells. The percentage of NG2$^+$/BrdU$^+$ related to the total number of NG2 cells was significantly increased after SCI (*** $p < 0.001$ vs. CTL). PROG further increased this percentage as compared to SCI (* $p < 0.05$ vs. SCI). **b** Effects of SCI and PROG treatment on the co-localization of the mature oligodendrocyte marker CC1 with bromodeoxyuridine (BrdU). Results represent the number of CC1$^+$ cells/0.1 mm^2. Open bars indicate the number of CC1$^+$/BrdU$^-$ cells whereas dark bars represent the number of CC1$^+$/BrdU$^+$. The number of CC1$^+$ cells was significantly decreased after SCI ($^{++}$ $p < 0.01$ vs. CTL) and restored after PROG treatment ($^{+++}$ $p < 0.001$ vs. SCI). Most cells did not show BrdU staining (dark bars) in CTL and SCI groups. However, after PROG treatment the number of CC1$^+$/BrdU$^+$ cells represents almost half of the total CC1$^+$ population (** $p < 0.01$ vs. CTL, SCI).

counted in dorsal, ventral and lateral white tracts of the spinal cord.

Three and 21 days after the lesion, we found that SCI produces a significant increase in the number of OPC in all white matter tracts, which were almost absent in control animals. These recruitment, however, was concomitant with a dramatic depletion of the total number of mature oligodendrocytes CC1$^+$ (fig. 1b), a decreased expression of the basic myelin protein (MBP), proteolipid protein (PLP) and myelin transcription factors [8] suggesting ongoing demyelination. Interestingly, 3 days after PROG administration we observed that OPC cell density was further increased over vehicle-treated animals, as well as the levels of expression of MBP and the transcription factors Olig2 and Nkx2.2, responsible to induce differentiation of OPC into mature forms. However, at 21 days after PROG treatment the early rise of OPC promoted by the steroid falls down and is coincident with an increase in the number of mature CC1$^+$ oligodendrocytes (fig. 1b), suggesting differentiation of OPC.

Thus, two interesting questions evolve from this scenario: (1) Does PROG stimulate the early proliferation of OPC? (2) Does PROG induce the differentiation of early proliferating OPC into mature oligodendrocytes?

In order to assess whether PROG had stimulated the proliferation of OPC during the 3-day period, the effects of injury and steroid treatment were studied by co-localizing of bromodeoxyuridine (BrdU) labeling with the NG2 marker. Three days after injury, as illustrated in figure 1a, the percentage of NG2$^+$/BrdU$^+$ cells related to NG2 total cell number was significantly increased in the SCI group. Interestingly, steroid administration further increased the number of double-labeled cells, supporting the notion that in this time-period PROG administration enhances the proliferation of OPC.

To answer the second question, we studied the presence of the BrdU marker into mature oligodendrocyte cells by confocal microscopy. BrdU was administered during 2 and 3 days after SCI and the number of CC1$^+$/BrdU$^+$ and CC1$^+$/BrdU$^-$ cells was counted after 21 days postinjury. As previously mentioned, the total number of CC1$^+$ cells was dramatically decreased 21 days after SCI as compared to control animals ($^{++}$ $p < 0.01$ vs. CTL; fig. 1b) and further increased after PROG administration ($^{+++}$ $p < 0.001$ vs. SCI). Our experiments also revealed that most CC1$^+$ cells did not show BrdU staining in the control (CTL) and after SCI (fig. 1b, dark bars). However, a strong colocalization of both markers was obtained in the SCI+PROG group (** $p < 0.01$ vs. SCI; fig. 1b, dark bars), representing almost half of the total CC1$^+$ cells. These changes were accompanied by increased expression of PLP and transcription factor Olig1, which is required for oligodendrogenesis and to repair demyelinating lesions. In conclusion, our observations support the assumption that the observed increase in the total number of $CC1^+$ cells after PROG treatment was due to the enhanced differentiation of the early proliferating OPC into mature $CC1^+$ cells.

Mechanisms of Progesterone Action in the Spinal Cord

The spinal cord expresses an array of progesterone receptors (PR), including the classic nuclear receptors PR-A and PR-B, the newly cloned membrane receptors mPR and the membrane-associated protein PGRMC1 [6, 9], that support the possibility of direct and multiple mechanisms of action in this tissue. Furthermore, non-nuclear-mediated actions derive from the rapid conversion of PROG into its reduced metabolites [10], which also display neuroactive properties. Since PROG offers a promising therapeutic perspective after central trauma or disease, the contributions to unravel its mechanisms of action remain an expanding and interesting field of research with potential clinical connotations [6].

Concluding Remarks

Data summarized here indicate that spinal cord injury provides a permissive environment for neuroactive steroid action. PROG significantly enhances BDNF neuronal expression, prevents the injury-induced chromatolytic changes of spinal neurons and stimulates the expression of key enzymes for the normal neuronal metabolism and neurotransmission. In addition, this steroid becomes a promyelinating factor, by stimulating the proliferation and differentiation of oligodendrocyte progenitors and myelin proteins synthesis. Thus, our observations further support the role of PROG as a promising therapeutic agent for the treatment of spinal cord injury and/or neurodegenerative diseases.

Acknowledgements

The authors acknowledge the support of the University of Buenos Aires (M808, M611), the National Research Council of Argentina (CONICET, PIP 5542) and FONCYT (BID 1728 OC AR/PICT 2006 No. 00291).

References

1 Bareyre FM, Schwab ME: Inflammation, degeneration and regeneration in the injured spinal cord: insights from DNA microarrays. Trends Neurosci 2003;26:555–563.
2 Nacimiento W, Sappok T, Brook GA, Tóth L, Schoen SW, Noth J, Kreutzberg GW: Structural changes of anterior horn neurons and their synaptic input caudal to low thoracic spinal cord hemisection in the adult rat: a light and electron microscopic study. Acta Neuropathol 1995;90:552–564.
3 Labombarda F, González SL, González-Deniselle MC, Guennoun R, Schumacher M, De Nicola AF: Cellular basis for progesterone neuroprotection in the injured spinal cord. J of Neurotrauma 2002;19:343–355.
4 González SL, Labombarda F, Gonzalez Deniselle MC, Mougel A, Guennoun R, Schumacher M, De Nicola AF: Progesterone neuroprotection in spinal cord trauma involves up-regulation of brain-derived neurotrophic factor in motoneurones. J Steroid Biochem Mol Biol 2005;94:143–149.
5 González SL, López Costa JJ, Labombarda MF, Gonzalez Deniselle MC, Guennoun R, Schumacher M, De Nicola AF: Progesterone effects on neuronal ultrastructure and expression of microtubule-associated protein 2 (MAP2) in rats with acute spinal cord injury. Cell Mol Neurobiol 2009;29:27–39.
6 De Nicola AF, Labombarda F, González Deniselle MC, González SL, Garay L, Meyer M, Gargiulo G, Guennoun R, Schumacher M: Progesterone neuroprotection in traumatic CNS injury and motoneuron degeneration. Front Neuroendocrinol 2009;30:173–187.
7 Jodhka PK, Kaur P, Underwood W, Lydon JP, Singh M: The differences in neuroprotective efficacy of progesterone and medroxyprogesterone acetate correlate with their effects on brain-derived neurotrophic factor expression. Endocrinology 2009;150:3162–3168.
8 Labombarda MF, Gonzalez SL, Lima A, Roig P, Guennoun R, Schumacher M, De Nicola AF: Effects of progesterone on oligodendrocyte progenitors, oligodendrocyte transcription factors, and myelin proteins following spinal cord injury. Glia 2009;57:884–897.
9 Labombarda F, González SL, González Deniselle MC, Vinson GP, Schumacher M, De Nicola AF, Guennoun R: Effects of injury and progesterone treatment on progesterone receptor and progesterone binding protein 25-DX expression in the rat spinal cord. J Neurochem 2003;87:902–913.
10 Labombarda F, Pianos A, Liere P, Eychenne B, González S, Cambourg A, De Nicola AF, Schumacher M, Guennoun R: Injury elicited increase in spinal cord neurosteroid content analyzed by gas chromatography mass spectrometry. Endocrinology 2006;147:1847–1859.

NeuroImmunoModulation

Neuroimmunomodulation 2010;17:150–152
DOI: 10.1159/000258710

Published online: February 4, 2010

Inflammatory Agents Involved in Septic Miscarriage

Julieta Aisemberg Claudia Vercelli Manuel Wolfson Ana Inés Salazar
Claudia Osycka-Salut Silvia Billi María Laura Ribeiro Mariana Farina
Ana María Franchi

Laboratory of Physiopathology of Pregnancy and Labor – Center for Pharmacological and Botanical Studies (CEFYBO, CONICET), School of Medicine, University of Buenos Aires, Buenos Aires, Argentina

Key Words
Pregnancy · Sepsis · Miscarriage · Nitric oxide · Endocannabinoids · Prostaglandins

Abstract
Even though the understanding of the cause of early pregnancy loss due to chromosomal abnormalities has improved, there is a dearth of knowledge of the causes of loss in euploid conceptuses. Maternal infections are a cause of abort in humans, but the mechanisms are not clear, so we have developed a murine model to study the mechanism of septic abortion by inducing embryonic resorption (ER) with lipopolysaccharide (LPS). We demonstrated that augmented production of nitric oxide (NO) and prostaglandins (PG) is involved in ER, and that inhibitors of their synthesis could prevent ER. Also, we observed an increase in the oxidative damage, evidenced by nitration of tyrosine proteins, due to the peroxynitrite anion. Since an association between chronic marijuana smoking and early miscarriage has been shown in women, we studied the participation of anandamide (AEA), the principal endocannabinoid, on the mechanism of action of LPS. We showed that LPS-induced NO synthesis and tissue damage were mediated by AEA, and that this endotoxin inhibited AEA degradation and increased its synthesis. These results suggest that several inflammatory molecules participate in the mechanism of early pregnancy loss and that their modulation could be useful tools to prevent it.

Most relevant studies in animals and humans indicate that some degree of systemic or uterine inflammation is necessary both for normal implantation and pregnancy. However, if inflammation becomes excessive, it might cause pregnancy complications such as fetal resorption/miscarriage. Genital tract bacterial infections could induce abortion and are some of the most common complications of pregnancy; however, the mechanisms remain unclear [1].

During early pregnancy in mice, the implantation sites are highly sensitive to proinflammatory molecules such as lipopolysaccharide (LPS) and Th1 cytokines (IFN-γ, TNF-α and IL-2). It has been reported that these molecules are capable of inducing embryonic resorption [2]. In early pregnancy, low doses of LPS that reproduce most of the systemic and cellular effects of sepsis, without affecting maternal survival, produce high percentage of embryonic resorption (ER) [3].

We investigated the role of several inflammatory agents in the mechanism of LPS-induced pregnancy loss in a mouse model.

NO is an important regulator of the biology and physiology of the organs of the reproductive system, including the uterus. Myometrial smooth muscle cells express eNOS (endothelial NO synthase), and the uterus is included in the list of 'tissue exceptions' and thus expresses iNOS (inducible NOS) even under unstimulated conditions [4].

KARGER
Fax +41 61 306 12 34
E-Mail karger@karger.ch
www.karger.com

© 2010 S. Karger AG, Basel
1021–7401/10/0173–0150$26.00/0

Accessible online at:
www.karger.com/nim

Ana María Franchi
Center for Pharmacological and Botanical Studies (CEFYBO, CONICET)
Paraguay 2155, Buenos Aires 1121 (Argentina)
Tel. +54 11 4508 3680, int. 111, Fax +54 11 4508 3680, int. 106
E-Mail afranchi@mail.retina.ar

It is well known that NO fulfills important functions during pregnancy; however, in high concentrations it could exert toxic effects since it works as a free radical. In the murine model of embryonic resorption the treatment with LPS increased decidual and uterine NO production, and this increase is due to the induction of iNOS isoform expression in decidua and uterus, and nNOS isoform expression only in decidua. LPS also caused fibrinolysis and infiltration of mesometrial decidua by positive iNOS macrophages [3].

Aminoguanidine (AG), an inhibitor of iNOS activity, reversed the LPS-induced embryonic resorption. This could be explained by an inhibition of the increase in NO production but also by an inhibition of the cellular infiltration and fibrinolysis. The effect of AG reverting the embryonic resorption and standardizing NOS activity suggests that NO participates in the process of embryonic resorption induced by LPS.

Prostaglandins mediate septisemic signs and symptoms [5] and stimulate myometrium contractility, so they could be abortifacients and are likely to be important mediators of LPS-induced embryonic resorption.

PG synthesis was stimulated under septic conditions in uterus and deciduas in a murine model of embryonic resorption due to LPS [6], and the administration of cyclooxygenase (COX) inhibitors showed that COX-II was the principal isoform involved in PG augmented synthesis [6]. Although COX-II mRNA expression and PG synthesis were stimulated in the uterus, COX-II protein was not increased after LPS treatment as would be expected [6]. One possible explanation is that under septic conditions, NO-derived species could specifically modulate COX expression. In this sense nitration of COX-II tyrosine residues after LPS administration has been detected, suggesting that LPS might induce a rapid nitration of uterine COX-II protein [6]. This result is in accordance with the reported 'peroxide tone' [7] necessary for COX activation. Strong evidence indicates that peroxynitrite increases COX activity [7]. So, the stimulatory effect of LPS on PG synthesis is likely to be the result of peroxynitrite functioning as a peroxide activator of PG signaling [6].

Endocannabinoids are an emerging class of lipid mediators isolated from brain and peripheral tissues. A major endocannabinoid, anandamide (AEA), is an endogenous agonist of cannabinoid receptors that binds to both brain (CB1) and peripheral (CB2) cannabinoid receptors, thus mimicking some of the psychotropic, hypnotic, tranquilizing and analgesic effects of Δ9-tetrahydrocannabinol (THC, psychoactive principle of hashish and marijuana). AEA has a role in implantation and embryo development. However, high levels of this molecule correlate with fetal weight loss and abortion. Additionally, there is a strong association between chronic marijuana smoking and early miscarriage in women [8], and indeed THC has been shown to adversely affect the course and outcome of pregnancy in several animal studies [10]. Moreover, it has been shown that decreased activity and protein expression of fatty acid amide hydrolase (FAAH) in peripheral lymphocytes is an early marker (at 7 to 8 weeks of gestation) of miscarriage [8]. After being transported into the cell, AEA is subsequently broken down into arachidonic acid (AA) and ethanolamine by an endoplasmic reticular integral membrane-bound enzyme called FAAH [8].

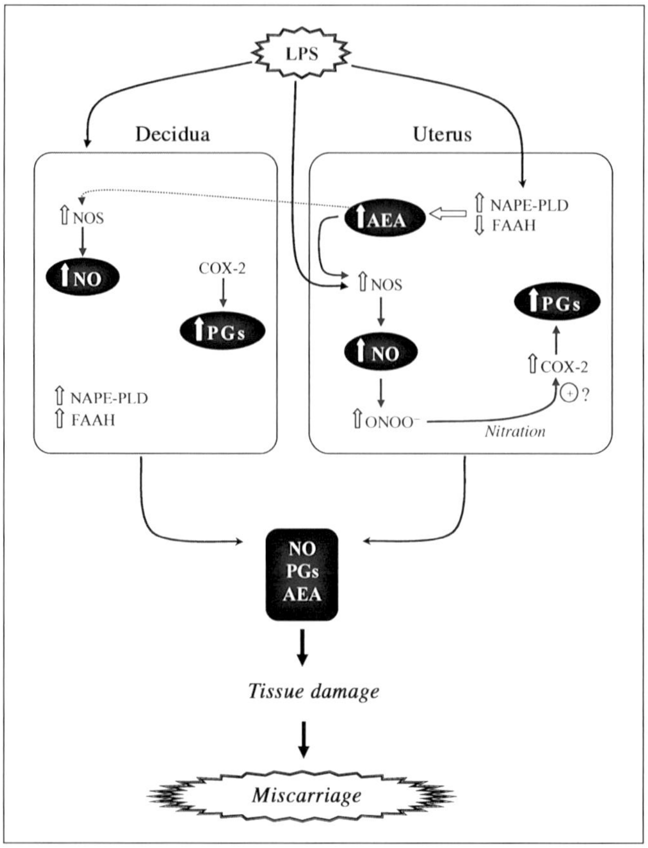

Fig. 1. LPS increased decidual and uterine NO production and induced NOS. The stimulatory effect of LPS on PG synthesis could be the result of peroxynitrite functioning as a peroxide activator of COX-2. LPS-induced NO production was mediated by AEA. LPS could be increasing AEA levels by inhibiting uterine FAAH activity and augmenting uterine and decidual NAPE-PLD expression. AEA could exert some positive effect on uterine and decidual NO production.

The uterus contains the highest concentrations of AEA yet discovered in mammalian tissues [8], and this suggests that it might play a role in reproduction. Anandamide can be generated from its membrane precursor N-arachidonoyl phosphatidylethanolamine (NAPE) through cleavage by a phospholipase D (NAPE-PLD, one of its synthesizing enzymes). Uterine AEA levels fluctuate with the state of pregnancy: downregulation of its levels is associated with uterine receptivity, while upregulation has been shown to impair pregnancy and embryo development in mice [8] and is correlated with uterine refractoriness to embryo implantation [8].

We evaluated if AEA participates in the mechanism of LPS-induced NO production on early murine pregnancy. For this purpose uterine and decidual explants were incubated in the presence of metha-anandamide (m-AEA, a stable analog of AEA). We observed that this stable synthetic AEA analog was able to induce NO production and iNOS protein expression. To confirm that AEA was modulating NO levels via iNOS, tissues were incubated in the presence of m-AEA plus 1,400 W (a selective iNOS inhibitor). We observed that NO production induced by m-AEA was markedly reduced by co-incubation of m-AEA with 1,400 W [9, 10]. Since m-AEA was also capable of inducing NO production, we examined whether LPS-induced NO production was mediated by AEA. Our results showed that decidual and uterine LPS-induced NO production was abrogated by co-incubation with CB1 (AM251) antagonist, which suggests that AEA is mediating LPS effect [9, 10].

On the other hand, we evaluated the contribution of LPS to AEA production by assessing the protein expression of NAPE-PLD in both tissues and we found that the endotoxin was able to induce a significant increase in NAPE-PLD expression [9, 10].

We have also analyzed whether LPS could modulate FAAH activity and expression. Here, we observed a tissue-specific reaction: LPS treatment increased decidual FAAH activity and protein expression, whereas the endotoxin decreased FAAH activity and expression in uterine explants [9, 10].

In mice the endometrial stroma undergoes dramatic cytologic changes to form a decidua in response to the implanting embryo. After attachment, the embryo becomes embedded in an enlarging mass of decidual tissue which remains very close to uterine tissue. Such proximity allows molecules to flow freely from one tissue to the other. Although we did not determine AEA levels, all this evidence led us to hypothezise that LPS could be increasing AEA levels by inhibiting uterine FAAH activity and augmenting uterine and decidual NAPE-PLD expression. Thus, even though LPS increased decidual FAAH activity, remaining AEA levels could still be exerting some effect on NO production. Furthermore, LPS induced tissue damage and this deleterious effect was partially abrogated by incubating tissue explants with LPS plus a CB1 receptor antagonist [9, 10]. These findings suggest that AEA, probably by increasing NO synthesis, participates in the deleterious effect of LPS in the implantation sites. The finding of an increase in nitrated proteins due to LPS could contribute to this hypothesis (fig. 1).

To date, an effective therapeutic does not exist to prevent early pregnancy loss. In this sense, these results suggest that several inflammatory molecules could participate in the mechanism of LPS-induced embryonic resorption and that their modulation by different NOS and COX inhibitors could be useful therapeutic agents to prevent this pathology.

References

1 Romero R, Roslansky P, Oyarzun E, Wan M, Emamian M, Novitsky TJ, Gould MJ, Hobbins JC: Labor and infection. II. Bacterial endotoxin in amniotic fluid and its relationship to the onset of preterm labor. Am J Obstet Gynecol 1988;158:1044.

2 Chaouat G, Menu E, Clark DA, Dy M, Minkowski M, Wegmann TG: Control of fetal survival in CBA × DBA/2 mice by lymphokine therapy. J Reprod Fertil 1990;89:447–458.

3 Ogando DG, Paz D, Cella M, Franchi AM: The fundamental role of increased production of nitric oxide in lipopolysaccharide-induced embryonic resorption in mice. Reproduction 2003;125:95.

4 Nakaya Y, Yamamoto S, Hamada Y, Kamada M, Aono T, Niwa M: Inducible nitric oxide synthase in uterine smooth muscle. Life Sci 1996;59:249.

5 Bone RC: Sepsis syndrome: new insights into its pathogenesis and treatment. Infect Dis Clin North Am 1991;5:793.

6 Aisemberg J, Vercelli C, Billi S, Ogando D, Ribeiro ML, Meiss R, McCann S, Rettori V, Franchi AM: Nitric oxide mediates prostaglandins' deleterious effect on lipopolysaccharide-triggered murine fetal resorption. Proc Natl Acad Sci USA 2007;104:7534.

7 Beharka AA, Wu D, Serafini M, Meydani SN: Mechanism of vitamin E inhibition of cyclooxygenase activity in macrophages from old mice: role of peroxynitrite. Free Radic Biol Med 2002;32:503.

8 Maccarrone M: Endocannabinoids: friends and foes of reproduction. Prog Lipid Res 2009;48:344–354.

9 Vercelli CA, Aisemberg J, Billi S, Cervini M, Ribeiro ML, Farina M, Franchi AM: Anandamide regulates lipopolysaccharide-induced nitric oxide synthesis and tissue damage in the murine uterus. Reprod Biomed Online 2009;18:824–831.

10 Vercelli CA, Aisemberg J, Billi S, Wolfson ML, Franchi AM: Endocannabinoid system and nitric oxide are involved in the deleterious effects of lipopolysaccharide on murine decidua. Placenta 2009;30:579–584.

NeuroImmunoModulation

Neuroimmunomodulation 2010;17:153–156
DOI: 10.1159/000258711

Published online: February 4, 2010

Endocannabinoid System Participates in Neuroendocrine Control of Homeostasis

Andrea De Laurentiis Javier Fernández Solari Claudia Mohn
María Zorrilla Zubilete Valeria Rettori

Centro de Estudios Farmacológicos y Botánicos, CEFYBO-CONICET-UBA, Facultad de Medicina, Universidad de Buenos Aires, Buenos Aires, Argentina

Key Words
Oxytocin · Vasopressin · Cannabinoid receptors · Nitric oxide · Hypothalamus · Neurohypophysis

Abstract
The hypothalamo-neurohypophyseal system plays a role in homeostasis under a variety of stress conditions, including endotoxemia. Oxytocin (OXT) and vasopressin (VP) are important hormones synthesized by neurons in the hypothalamic paraventricular and supraoptic nuclei and released into different brain regions and from the neurohypophyseal terminals into the blood in response to many patho-physiological stimuli. However, the mechanism that controls OXT and VP secretion has not been fully elucidated. Nitric oxide (NO) is a known mediator that regulates the release of these hormones. The endocannabinoid system is a new intercellular system that modulates several neuroendocrine actions. Endocannabinoids (eCB) are released as retrograde messengers by many neurons, including hypothalamic magnocellular neurons and cannabinoid receptors are localized within these neurons, as well as in the anterior and posterior pituitary lobes, suggesting an eCB role in the production and release of OXT and VP. Lipopolysaccharide (LPS) injection is a model used as immune challenge. LPS causes a neuroendocrine response that is mediated by cytokines, tumor necrosis factor-α being one of them. We focused on NO and endocannabinoid system participation on OXT and VP production and secretion during basal and stress conditions and found that eCB affect basal OXT and VP secretion by acting differently at each level of the hypothalamo-neurohypophyseal system. After LPS, there is an increase in eCB synthesis that enhances OXT secretion.

The hypothalamic-neurohypophyseal system is a neuroendocrine system essential for survival. It consists of the hypothalamic supraoptic nuclei (SON) situated lateral to the optic chiasm, and the paraventricular nuclei (PVN) on each side of the third ventricle. Magnocellular neurons in those nuclei synthesise oxytocin (OXT) and vasopressin (VP) and send axonal projections to the posterior pituitary. The neuronal activity stimulates the release of hormones into the blood, regulating a number of important physiological functions, mainly reproduction and homeostasis. In addition, OXT and VP have been shown to have neurotransmitter functions in various regions of the central nervous system (CNS), thus controlling complex neuroadaptive processes [1].

The endocannabinoid system has been recognized as a major neuromodulatory system, whose function is to maintain brain homeostasis. Endocannabinoids (eCB) are lipophilic arachidonic acid derivatives produced in

KARGER
Fax +41 61 306 12 34
E-Mail karger@karger.ch
www.karger.com

1021–7401/10/0173–0153$26.00/0

Accessible online at:
www.karger.com/nim

Dr. Andrea De Laurentiis, Centro de Estudios Farmacológicos y Botánicos (CEFYBO-CONICET-UBA), Facultad de Medicina, Universidad de Buenos Aires
Paraguay 2155, piso 16, Buenos Aires ABG1121 (Argentina)
Tel. +54 11 4508 3680, int. 112, Fax +54 11 4508 3680, int. 106
E-Mail andredelaurentiis@yahoo.com

brain and peripheral tissues. Several eCB have been identified. The first discovered, and more studied endogenous ligand for cannabinoid receptors is anandamide (AEA). Anandamide formation via energy-independent condensation of arachidonic acid and ethanolamine is attributed to an enzymatic activity termed 'anandamide synthase'. It has been proposed that this reaction is catalized by fatty acid amide hydrolase (FAAH), the enzyme that hydrolyzes AEA acting in reverse. Another pathway of AEA biosynthesis involves the hydrolysis of a phospholipid precursor catalyzed by phospholipase D. Depolarization of the postsynaptic cells generates eCB that act retrogradely to inhibit subsequent neurotransmitter release by its binding to a seven transmembrane $G_{i/o}$-coupled cannabinoid receptors. Two subtypes of cannabinoid (CB) receptors, CB_1 and CB_2, have been identified and cloned. The CB_1 receptor is the predominant subtype in the CNS, whereas the CB_2 receptor is primarily expressed in immune cells, although it is also found in glial cells of the CNS [2]. The eCB have affinity not only for CB_1 and CB_2 receptors, but also for the transient potential vanilloid type 1 receptor (TRPV1). Anandamide is involved through TRPV1 in physiological processes such as blood pressure control, pain sensation and airway responsiveness [8]. The eCB action is terminated by its removal from the extracellular space. The eCB are transported across the cell membrane by a cannabinoid transporter and degraded by the enzyme FAAH.

Recent reports have highlighted the interaction between the endocannabinoid system and the modulation of the physiology of magnocellular neurons, since OXT and eCB cooperate to shape the electrophysiological properties of SON neurons [1]. To date, most studies in this field focus on the relationship of these systems and their roles in the hypothalamus; however, there are no studies about the eCB action and function in the neurohypophysis (NH) to understand its participation in the regulation of OXT and VP release. By testing several concentrations of AEA (10^{-11} to 10^{-8} M), we have recently demonstrated that it decreases OXT and VP secretion in incubated neurohypophyses from adult male Sprague-Dawley rats, 10^{-9} M being the most effective inhibitory concentration.

Nitric oxide (NO) is a gaseous molecule and a highly reactive free radical produced from L-arginine by nitric oxide synthase (NOS) with multiple and complex roles within many biological systems. Although the involvement of NO in the regulation of OXT and VP release has been investigated, the complicated mechanisms involved remain unclear [3]. Neural NOS (nNOS) coexists with OXT and VP, not only in the cell bodies of hypothalamic magnocellular neurons but also in the axon terminals in the neural pituitary lobe. In our previous work, we demonstrated in vitro that NO donors reduce OXT secretion from the neural pituitary lobe [4] and that neurokinin A increases neurohypophyseal NOS activity. Therefore, this increased production of NO inhibits OXT secretion from this tissue [5]. Very recently, we confirmed that NO reduces both OXT and VP secretion from NH of male adult rats and thus studied the interrelation between the endocannabinoid system, NO and OXT/VP release. Our in vitro studies performed in tissues from untreated adult male rats showed that AEA increased NOS activity in the NH as well as in the hypothalamus. We also found that the inhibitory effect of AEA on OXT and VP secretion from the NH seems to be mediated by NO since the scavenging of NO by hemoglobin or the inhibition of NOS by L-NAME completely blocked this inhibitory effect.

Little is known about the expression and function of cannabinoid receptors in the posterior pituitary lobe. In this study, we performed pharmacological experiments in vitro in which the NH was incubated in the presence of AEA and cannabinoid or vanilloid receptor-selective antagonists. We found that the CB_2 and TRPV1 antagonists, AM630 and capsazepine, respectively, completely blocked the inhibitory effects of AEA on OXT and VP release from the NH. However, in the presence of CB_1 antagonist (AM251), the inhibitory effect of AEA persisted, suggesting that this subtype of cannabinoid receptor does not participate in OXT and VP release. These results indicate that AEA acts through CB_2 and TRPV1 receptors to inhibit the release of both neuropeptides at the neurohypophyseal level.

Stress is a response of an organism to challenges (stressors) from the environment, aimed at re-establishing homeostasis. In general, infection and inflammation are considered physical stressors. In response to them, hypothalamic neurons trigger the release of corticotrophin-releasing hormone (CRH) which leads to the activation of the hypothalamic-pituitary-adrenal axis. Besides CRH, other neuropeptides such as OXT and VP may act as secretagogues of adrenocorticotropic hormone (ACTH). These peptides act synergistically with CRH to stimulate ACTH release from the pituitary and therefore stimulate the adrenal gland. Recent data suggest that eCB may play a pivotal role in the regulation of this axis activity at hypothalamic level [2].

During infection, bacterial products such as lipopolysaccharide (LPS) cause the release of proinflammatory cytokines from immune cells. Also, LPS causes changes in the CNS, many of which are mediated by LPS-induced cytokine production in the brain, resulting in metabolic changes, induction of fever, etc. The neuroendocrine response to infection can be mimicked by peripheral injection of LPS, which is a commonly used model of immune challenge [6].

In a previous work, we demonstrated the connection between the immune and the endocannabinoid systems at the hypothalamic level by showing the increase of AEA synthase activity in hypothalami obtained from adult male rats injected i.p. with LPS [7]. It is known that tumor necrosis factor-α (TNF-α) is one of the main cytokines that mediate the effects attributed to LPS on the hypothalamic pituitary axis. The i.c.v. administration of TNF-α and the incubation of hypothalamic fragments with this cytokine also increase AEA synthase activity [7]. In addition, we have recently evaluated the in vitro effect of AEA on OXT production in hypothalamic fragments from untreated adult male rats. To this end, we incubated hypothalamic fragments containing SON and PVN nuclei in the presence of AEA (10^{-6} to 10^{-9} M) and observed that the lowest concentration tested significantly increased OXT production. This result is contrary to that observed in the NH. We also observed that the incubation with TNF-α increased OXT production from hypothalamic fragments and that this effect was mediated by endocannabinoids since the presence of CB_1 antagonist (AM251) completely blocked this effect (fig. 1).

It is known that LPS activates magnocellular OXT and VP neurons in SON and PVN; however, little is known about the participation of the endocannabinoid system in this effect. Additionally, we performed in vivo experiments where adult male rats received a single i.p. dose of LPS. We observed that LPS i.p. injection increased plasma OXT and TNF-α levels after 1 h of administration, returning to basal levels at 3 h post injection. Blockade of hypothalamic cannabinoid receptors CB_1 and CB_2 by i.c.v. administration of selective antagonists, AM251 and AM630 respectively, attenuated the LPS-induced increases in plasma OXT and TNF-α levels. Also, enhancing hypothalamic endocannabinoid signaling by i.c.v. administration of a FAAH inhibitor (URB597) potentiated LPS-induced increases in circulating OXT and TNF-α levels. The amplification of endocannabinoid signaling at the hypothalamic level thus seems to facilitate the response of neuropeptides and cytokines after an acute immune challenge. These recent results suggest that endocannabinoids may signal through hypothalamic cannabinoid receptors to facilitate LPS-induced neuroendocrine response during infection and are in concordance with previous works of others [9] (fig. 1).

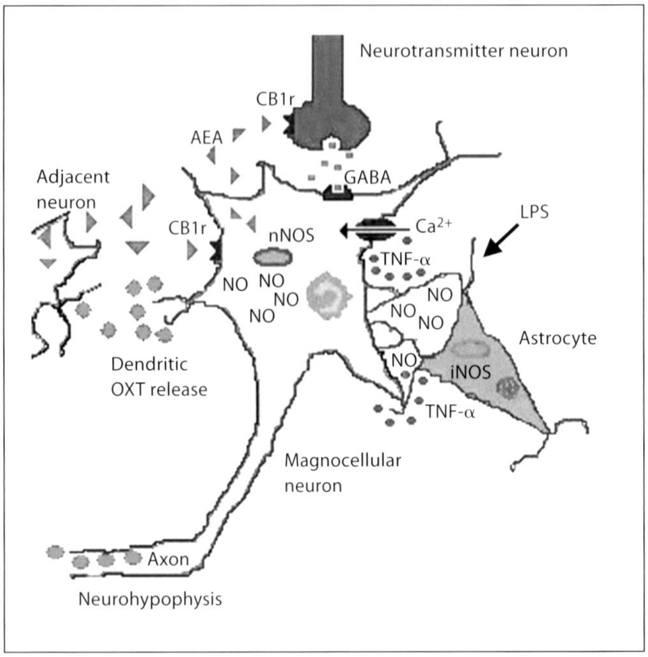

Fig. 1. Postulated mechanism for endocannabinoid participation in OXT release from PVN and SON hypothalamic nuclei after LPS challenge: LPS challenge increases the brain production of cytokines, between them TNF-α. There is also iNOS activation from astrocytes with an increase in NO production. These factors and Ca^{2+} depolarization induce the activation of magnocellular neurons increasing the release of OXT. Also, LPS increase the synthesis of AEA which stimulates nNOS activity, increasing NO stimulating OXT release. Furthermore, AEA acts as a retrograde messenger on CB_1 receptors present on presynaptic terminals of adjacent neurons. Since CB_1 are $G_{i/o}$-coupled receptors, AEA inhibition of inhibitory GABA adds to the augmentation of OXT release.

In our studies, we focused on the participation of NO and the endocannabinoid system on OXT and VP production and secretion during basal and stress conditions.

Our results are in agreement with most of the data in the literature since it is well known that cannabinoids exert inhibitory effects on hormone secretion from pituitary gland having inhibitory impact on neuroendocrine function. One notable exception to this cannabinoid inhibition of hypothalamic neuroendocrine function is the reported stimulatory effect of cannabinoids on the stress-induced hypothalamic pituitary adrenal axis. Activation of the axis is the main neuroendocrine response to stress and cannabinoids, rather than suppressing this axis, have been shown to enhance secretion of hypothalamic-pituitary hormones.

The results were assessed by modulating NO and endocannabinoid signaling by pharmacological means and sometimes differed depending at which level we performed the in vitro experiments. We consider that the results obtained in the in vivo model of LPS challenge show a real landscape of the situation since the hypothalamo-pituitary-adrenal axis is influenced by many neuroimmunoendocrine signals.

In summary, the present results are in agreement with the fact that the endocannabinoid system of the brain plays an important role in homeostasis by regulating hypothalamo-neurohypophyseal axis activity.

Acknowledgments

The present work was supported by the grants from Consejo Nacional de Investigaciones Científicas y Técnicas (CONICET) PIP 6149 and PIP 02546 and Agencia Nacional de Promoción Científica y Tecnológica PICT 06-0258.

References

1 McDonald NA, Kuzmiski JB, Naderi N, Schwab Y, Pittman QJ: Endogenous modulators of synaptic transmission: cannabinoid regulation in the supraopitc nucleus; in Neumann ID, Landgraf R (eds): Progress in Brain Research. Oxford, Elsevier, 2008, vol 170, pp 129–136.

2 Steiner MA, Wotjak CT: Role of the endocannabinoid system in regulation of the hypothalamic-pituitary-adrenocortical axis; in Neumann ID, Landgraf R (eds): Progress in Brain Research. Oxford, Elsevier, 2008, vol 170, pp 397–432.

3 Rettori V, Fernandez-Solari J, Mohn C, Zorrilla Zubilete MA, de la Cal C, Prestifilippo JP, De Laurentiis A: Nitric oxide at the crossroad of immunoneuroendocrine interactions. Ann NY Acad Sci 2009;1153:35–47.

4 Rettori V, Canteros G, Reynoso R, Gimeno M, McCann SM: Oxytocin stimulates the release of luteinizing hormone-releasing hormone from medial basal hypothalamic explants by releasing nitric oxide. Proc Natl Acad Sci USA 1997;94:2741–2744.

5 De Laurentiis A, Pisera D, Duvilanski B, Rettori V, Lasaga M, Seilicovich A: Neurokinin A inhibits oxytocin and GABA release from GABA release from the posterior pituitary by stimulating nitric oxide synthase. Brain Res Bull 2000;53:325–330.

6 McCann SM, Antunes Rodrigues J, Franci CR, Anselmo-Franci JA, Karanth S, Rettori V: Role of the hypothalamic pituitary adrenal axis in the control of the response to stress and infection. Braz J Med Biol Res 2000;33:1121–1131.

7 Fernandez-Solari J, Prestifilippo JP, Bornstein SR, McCann SM, Rettori V: Participation of the endocannabinoid system in the effect of TNF-alpha on hypothalamic release of gonadotropin-releasing hormone. Ann NY Acad Sci 2006;1088:238–250.

8 van der Stelt M, Di Marzo V: Endovanilloids: Putative endogenous ligands of transient receptor potential vanilloid 1 channels. Eur J Biochem 2004;271:1827–1834.

9 Roche M, Kelly JP, O'Driscoll M, Finn DP: Augmentation of endogenous cannabinoid tone modulates lipopolysaccharide-induced alterations in circulating cytokine levels in rats. Immunology 2008;125:263–271.

NeuroImmunoModulation

Neuroimmunomodulation 2010;17:157–160
DOI: 10.1159/000258712

Published online: February 4, 2010

Tolerogenic Dendritic Cells in the Control of Autoimmune Neuroinflammation: An Emerging Role of Protein-Glycan Interactions

Juan M. Ilarregui[a] Gabriel A. Rabinovich[a, b]

[a]Laboratorio de Inmunopatología, Instituto de Biología y Medicina Experimental, Consejo Nacional de Investigaciones Científicas y Técnicas, y [b]Departamento de Química Biológica, Facultad de Ciencias Exactas y Naturales, Universidad de Buenos Aires, Buenos Aires, Argentina

Key Words

Dendritic cells · Multiple sclerosis · Neuroinflammation · Experimental autoimmune encephalomyelitis · Galectin-1 · Interleukin-27 · Interleukin-10

Abstract

During the past decade, a great deal of information has contributed to our understanding of the immunosuppressive pathways that operate during the resolution of autoimmune pathology, including central nervous system (CNS) inflammation. Activation of these pathways is accomplished through the integration of an intricate network of inhibitory signals and immune suppressive cells, including regulatory T cells, myeloid-derived suppressor cells, 'alternatively activated' macrophages and tolerogenic dendritic cells (DCs). During the course of inflammatory diseases, immature or mature DCs may be licensed by different stimuli (e.g. cytokines, neuropeptides and growth factors) to become tolerogenic and suppress pathogenic T cell responses, thus emphasizing the outstanding plasticity of these cells. Recent findings have shed light to an immunoregulatory circuit by which galectin-1, an endogenous glycan-binding protein, favors the differentiation of regulatory DCs which promote T cell tolerance and contribute to resolution of autoimmune pathology through mechanisms involving IL-27 and IL-10. Together with the ability of galectin-1-glycan interactions to selectively blunt T helper (Th)1 and Th17 responses, this effect provides a rational explanation for the broad immunosuppressive effects of this glycan-binding protein in several experimental models of chronic inflammation and cancer. In this mini review, we will summarize the regulatory signals leading to the differentiation of tolerogenic DCs and their participation in CNS inflammation. In addition, we will underscore recent findings on the emerging role of galectin-glycan interactions in the establishment of immunosuppressive networks during the resolution of chronic inflammation.

Dendritic Cells at the Crossroads of Tolerance and Inflammation

During the past years great progress has been made in our understanding of the cellular and molecular pathways that regulate immune tolerance [1]. Active immunosuppression can be achieved through the secretion of anti-inflammatory cytokines or through specialized suppressor cells, including $CD4^+CD25^+FoxP3^+$ T regulatory cells (T_{reg}) cells, type-1 $FoxP3^-$ T_{reg} cells, myeloid-derived suppressor cells, 'alternatively-activated' macrophages and tolerogenic dendritic cells (DCs) [1].

KARGER

Fax +41 61 306 12 34
E-Mail karger@karger.ch
www.karger.com

1021–7401/10/0173–0157$26.00/0

Accessible online at:
www.karger.com/nim

Dr. Gabriel A. Rabinovich, Instituto de Biología y Medicina Experimental (IBYME)
Consejo Nacional de Investigaciones Científicas y Técnicas (CONICET)
Vuelta de Obligado 2490, Ciudad de Buenos Aires C1428ADN (Argentina)
Tel. +54 11 4783 2869, ext. 236, Fax +54 11 4786 2564
E-Mail gabyrabi@gmail.com or gabyrabi@fibertel.com.ar

DCs are the central players in all immune responses, both innate and adaptive [1, 2]. Conventional DC subsets described in humans include myeloid DCs and plasmacytoid DCs [2]. Through antigen recognition, processing and presentation, DCs can orchestrate adaptive immune responses; yet these cells can also attenuate inflammatory reactions irrespective of their maturation status by promoting T cell anergy or favoring the expansion and/or differentiation of T_{reg} cells [2]. During the course of chronic inflammatory reactions, bidirectional interactions take place between dendritic cells (DCs) and T cells, which may initiate either an immunogenic or tolerogenic pathway [2]. Several stimuli may influence the decision of DCs to become tolerogenic, including transforming growth factor-β, interleukin (IL)-10, vasoactive intestinal peptide, hepatocyte growth factor, and 1,25-dihydroxyvitamin D_3 [1, 2]. In addition, interaction with stromal cells, $CD4^+CD25^+FoxP3^+$ T_{reg} cells or apoptotic cells may also drive the differentiation of tolerogenic DCs [2]. In spite of early observations assigning a predominant immunogenic and pro-inflammatory function to mature DCs (which express high levels of major histocompatibility complex II and costimulatory molecules CD80/CD86), recent evidence challenged this paradigm showing that DC maturation itself is neither an immunogenic nor a tolerogenic hallmark of DCs [2]. Supporting this concept, fully mature DCs are abundant throughout the peak and resolution phase of autoimmune inflammation and are capable of promoting the expansion of T_{reg} cells instead of inciting a primary or memory T cell response [1–3]. Hence, it is the flexibility of specialized DCs to respond to selective environmental signals, which may determine the amplification or silencing of Th1-, Th2-, Th17- or Th9-driven effector immunity, which may in turn shape the course of chronic inflammation. The mechanisms and pathways underlying these regulatory processes are subject of an intensive research with still more questions than answers.

Tolerogenic Dendritic Cells in CNS Autoimmune Inflammation

Multiple sclerosis is a major inflammatory and demyelinating disorder of the CNS characterized by a relapsing-remitting stage followed by a secondary progressive phase [3]. Animal models of experimental autoimmune encephalomyelitis (EAE) recapitulate the clinical and immunological features of the disease and have been of crucial importance for the validation of many therapeutic agents [3]. From an immunological standpoint, the activity of the disease is controlled through a delicate balance of Th1, Th2, Th17 and T_{reg} cells [3]. While DCs producing high amounts of IL-12 favor the differentiation of Th1 effector cells, IL-23-secreting DCs favor a Th17 pathogenic phenotype and those producing high amounts of IL-10 and IL-27 determine the differentiation of $FoxP3^-$ T_{reg} cells [1, 3, 4]. In this regard, alterations in DC activation and cytokine production have been shown to contribute to the transition from the relapsing-remitting to the progressive phase of multiple sclerosis [3]. Hence, targeting pro-inflammatory Th1 or Th17 effector cells, promoting the expansion of T_{reg} cells or fine-tuning the tolerogenic function of DCs have emerged as rational therapeutic strategies aimed at tempering autoimmune neuroinflammation and protecting the CNS from immune-mediated damage [3].

Galectin-Glycan Interactions in the Regulation of CNS Autoimmunity

Endogenous glycan-binding proteins or lectins control a variety of biological processes by deciphering information encoded by cell surface glycoproteins and glycolipids [4]. Galectins are a family of ubiquitous lectins defined by a conserved carbohydrate-recognition domain and a common structural fold [4]. Galectins preferentially bind to β-galactoside-containing glycans comprised of repeating units of N-acetyllactosamine (Galβ1,4GlcNAc), either as disaccharide units at the termini of complex N-glycans or as repeating units in a poly-N-acetyllactosamine chain on N-glycans or O-glycans [4]. As many as 15 galectins have been identified in mammals and proposed to mediate diverse biological roles in the regulation of innate and adaptive immune responses, including cytokine receptor endocytosis, host-pathogen interactions and homeostasis of immune cells [4]. Galectin-1, a prototype member of this family, can modulate T cell functions by controlling the proliferation and survival of effector T cells, antagonizing T cell activation or modulating the balance of pro-inflammatory and anti-inflammatory cytokines [4].

Compelling evidence indicates that galectin-1 treatment suppresses chronic inflammation and skews the balance of the immune responses towards a Th2-type cytokine profile in several experimental models of autoimmune inflammation, including arthritis, uveitis, inflammatory bowel disease, diabetes, hepatitis and autoimmune encephalomyelitis [reviewed in 4]. In addition, selective blockade of galectin-1 expression in tumor tis-

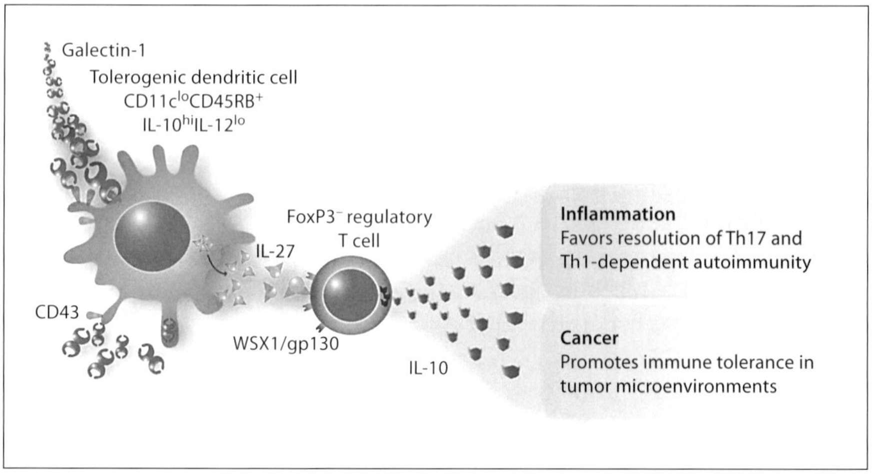

Color version available online

Fig. 1. Identification of an immunoregulatory circuit linking galectin-1 signaling, IL-27-producing DCs and IL-10-secreting T_{reg} cells. During the peak and resolution stages of autoimmune neuroinflammation, galectin-1 expression augments and promotes the differentiation of $CD11c^{lo}$, $CD45RB^{+}$ tolerogenic DCs which express high levels of phosphorylated STAT3 (pSTAT3) and IL-10. These DCs also secrete high amounts of IL-27, a heterodimeric cytokine composed of the p28 and the EBI3 subunits, which interacts with its specific receptor (gp130/WSX1) and promotes the expansion of IL-10-producing $FoxP3^{-}$ regulatory T cells. Delivery of these tolerogenic signals from dendritic cells to T cells blunt Th1 and Th17 responses and promote the resolution of autoimmune neuroinflammation. On the other hand, hierarchical expression of these immunoregulatory signals may contribute to create a tolerogenic microenvironment at sites of tumor growth, suggesting that targeting the gears of this tolerogenic circuit may have broad therapeutic implications in immunopathology.

sue results in reduced tumor growth and unleashed Th1-mediated antitumor responses in experimental settings of melanoma and Hodgkin lymphoma, suggesting the involvement of this glycan-binding protein in tumor-immune escape [5, 6]. Recent work provided a molecular explanation for galectin-1-mediated Th2 skewing, demonstrating that Th1 and Th17 effector cells express the repertoire of cell surface glycans that are essential for the formation of galectin-glycoprotein lattices, and hence are cellular targets of the immunoregulatory activity of galectin-1. By contrast, Th2 cells are protected from galectin-1 binding through differential α2,6 sialylation of cell surface glycoproteins [7]. Consistent with these findings, galectin-1-deficient *(Lgals1*$^{-/-}$*)* mice challenged with encephalitogenic stimuli developed greater antigen-specific Th1 and Th17 responses compared to their wild-type counterpart [7].

To further understand the cellular and molecular mechanisms underlying the broad immunosuppressive activity of galectin-1 in autoimmunity and tumor settings, we investigated the impact of this glycan-binding protein on human and mouse DCs using different experimental models in vivo [8]. Notably, DCs differentiated or matured in a galectin-1-enriched microenvironment acquired a distinctive 'regulatory signature' characterized by high expression of the cell surface marker CD45RB, phosphorylation of the transcription factor STAT3 and abundant secretion of IL-27 and IL-10 [8]. More importantly, when transferred in vivo, these DCs promoted T-cell tolerance in antigen-specific and neoplastic settings, blunted Th1 and Th17 responses and halted autoimmune neuroinflammation through mechanisms involving DC-derived IL-27 and T cell-derived IL-10 [8]. Thus, using IL-27 receptor-deficient *(Il27ra*$^{-/-}$*)* and IL-10-deficient *(Il10*$^{-/-}$*)* mice, we have identified an immunoregulatory circuit linking galectin-1 signaling, IL-27-producing tolerogenic DCs and IL-10 secreting T_{reg} cells (fig. 1) [8]. Interestingly, other studies have found that DCs engineered to overexpress galectin-1 can induce contrasting effects on naïve and stimulated T cells similar to direct exposure of T cells to soluble recombinant galectin-1 [9], suggesting that these cells could also be used as vehicles of immunomodulatory target genes. Moreover, exposure to galectin-1 also promoted the migration of DCs through mechanisms involving Syk and PKC signaling [10], suggesting that DCs exposed to galectin-1 may acquire a distinctive immunomodulatory program characterized by a 'mature' or 'semi-mature' cell surface phenotype, increased migration profile and greatly enhanced tolerogenic potential.

Given its tolerogenic effects, we also investigated the relevance of endogenous galectin-1 during the evolution of CNS autoimmune inflammation. Remarkably, galectin-1 expression augmented during the peak and recovery phases of EAE and was dramatically upregulated by tolerogenic stimuli including vasoactive intestinal peptide, vitamin D_3 and IL-10, but significantly downregulated by pro-inflammatory cytokines (TNF and IFN-γ) and most Toll-like receptor agonists [8]. Moreover, DCs lacking *Lgals1* gene had lower expression of IL-27, higher expression of IL-23 and less STAT3 phosphorylation and were not capable of promoting T cell tolerance during ongoing EAE [8]. In contrast, galectin-1-sufficient DCs restored T cell tolerance and contributed to the resolution of autoimmune neuroinflammation [8], suggesting a crucial role of endogenous galectin-1 in 'fine-tuning' the immunogenicity of DCs.

Conclusions and Future Directions

Research over the past decade has identified a number of upstream and downstream signaling events on DCs which can be manipulated in a selective manner to amplify either an immunogenic or a tolerogenic response [1–3]. In this context, tolerogenic DCs may be employed as 'Trojan horses' to propagate immune tolerance and silence CNS inflammation. Hence, galectin-1-differentiated DCs producing IL-27 can be harnessed to silence Th1- and Th17-mediated responses and promote the differentiation of IL-10-producing T_{reg} cells, suggesting a hierarchy of tolerogenic signals which may represent potential targets in T cell-mediated demyelinating disease. However, before galectin-based therapeutic strategies can be embraced, a more thorough understanding of the mechanisms underlying the function of galectin-glycan lattices is required, including the extent of redundancy in galectin functions in vivo and the regulation of galectin expression in healthy, inflamed and neoplastic tissue.

Acknowledgments

We thank all members of our laboratory for helpful discussions, particularly to D.O. Croci and M.A. Toscano for figure design. Research in the authors' laboratory is supported by grants from The National Agency for Promotion of Science and Technology (Argentina), Sales Foundation for Cancer Research (Argentina), National Council of Scientific and Technical Investigation (CONICET; Argentina), The Cancer Research Institute (USA) and Prostate Cancer Foundation (UK). G.A.R. is a member of the Scientific Career of CONICET and J.M.I. is a postdoctoral fellow of CONICET.

References

1 Rabinovich GA, Gabrilovich D, Sotomayor EM: Immunosuppressive strategies that are mediated by tumor cells. Annu Rev Immunol 2007;25:267–296.
2 Rutella S, Danese S, Leone G: Tolerogenic dendritic cells: cytokine modulation comes of age. Blood 2006,108:1435–1440.
3 Lopez-Diego RS, Weiner HL: Novel therapeutic strategies for multiple sclerosis – a multifaceted adversary. Nat Rev Drug Discov 2008;7:909–925.
4 Rabinovich GA, Toscano MA: Turning 'sweet' on immunity: galectin-glycan interactions in immune tolerance and inflammation. Nat Rev Immunol 2009;9:338–352.
5 Rubinstein N, Alvarez MJ, Zwirner NW, Toscano MA, Ilarregui JM, Bravo A, Mordoh J, Fainboim L, Podhajcer OL, Rabinovich GA: Targeted inhibition of galectin-1 gene expression in tumor cells results in heightened T cell-mediated rejection: a potential mechanism of tumor-immune privilege. Cancer Cell 2004;5:241–251.
6 Juszczynski P, Ouyang J, Monti S, Rodig SJ, Takeyama K, Abramson J, Chen W, Kutok JL, Rabinovich GA, Shipp MA: The AP1-dependent secretion of galectin-1 by Reed Sternberg cells fosters immune privilege in classical Hodgkin lymphoma. Proc Natl Acad Sci USA 2007;104:13134–13139.
7 Toscano MA, Bianco GA, Ilarregui JM, Croci DO, Correale J, Hernandez JD, Zwirner NW, Poirier F, Riley EM, Baum LG, Rabinovich GA: Differential glycosylation of TH1, TH2 and TH-17 effector cells selectively regulates susceptibility to cell death. Nat Immunol 2007;8:825–834.
8 Ilarregui JM, Croci DO, Bianco GA, Toscano MA, Salatino M, Vermeulen ME, Geffner JR, Rabinovich GA: Tolerogenic signals delivered by dendritic cells to T cells through a galectin-1-driven immunoregulatory circuit involving interleukin 27 and interleukin 10. Nat Immunol 2009;10:981–991.
9 Perone MJ, Larregina AT, Shufesky WJ, Papworth GD, Sullivan ML, Zahorchak AF, Stolz DB, Baum LG, Watkins SC, Thomson AW, Morelli AE: Transgenic galectin-1 induces maturation of dendritic cells that elicit contrasting responses in naïve and activated T cells. J Immunol 2006;176:7207–7220.
10 Fulcher JA, Chang MH, Wang S, Almazan T, Hashimi ST, Eriksson AU, Wen X, Pang M, Baum LG, Singh RR, Lee B: Galectin-1 co-clusters CD43/CD45 on dendritic cells and induces cell activation and migration through Syk and PKC signaling. J Biol Chem 2009;284:26860–26870.

NeuroImmunoModulation

Neuroimmunomodulation 2010;17:161–164
DOI: 10.1159/000258713

Published online: February 4, 2010

Keeping the Balance between Immune Tolerance and Pathogen Immunity with Endogenous Neuropeptides

Elena Gonzalez-Rey

Instituto de Parasitología y Biomedicina López-Neyra, CSIC, Granada, Spain

Key Words

Inflammation · Homeostasis · Antimicrobial peptides · Trypanosomatids

Abstract

Identification of the factors that regulate the immune tolerance and control the appearance of exacerbated inflammatory conditions is crucial for the development of new therapies of inflammatory and autoimmune diseases. Although much is known about the molecular basis of initiating signals and pro-inflammatory chemical mediators in inflammation, it has only recently become apparent that endogenous stop signals are critical at early checkpoints within the temporal events of inflammation. Some neuropeptides and hormones that are produced during the ongoing inflammatory response have emerged as endogenous anti-inflammatory agents that participate in the regulation of the processes that ensure self-tolerance and/or inflammation resolution. We will examine the latest research findings, which indicate that neuropeptides participate in maintaining immune tolerance in two distinct ways: by regulating the balance between pro-inflammatory and anti-inflammatory factors, and by inducing the emergence of regulatory T cells with suppressive activity against autoreactive T cell effectors. We will also examine the role of some of these neuropeptides as mediators of innate defense acting as natural antimicrobial peptides. Both anti-inflammatory and pro-resolving neuropeptides have shown therapeutic potential for a variety of inflammatory and autoimmune disorders and could be used as biotemplates for the development of novel pharmacologic agents. From a physiological point of view, neuropeptides play a critical role in the innate-adaptive immune cross talk that allows survival.

Living organisms are continuously being faced with pathogens. Survival requires immune protection against infection. Failure to establish or restore homeostatic conditions during or following the onset of an infection can lead to tissue damage and could induce harmful autoimmune responses. In this situation, immune cells and the molecules that respond to pathogen-derived antigens also react to self-antigens. Keeping the immune homeostasis is a daunting job for the immune system. The most important immune mechanisms that collaborate to ensure self-tolerance are central clonal deletion, effector T cell balance, regulatory T cells and cytokine deviation. In the last years, numerous researchers have focused on the identification of the endogenous factors involved in the regulation of immune balance. Some of the immunosuppressive cytokines such as IL-10 and transforming growth factor-β1 have demonstrated to have this role. However,

KARGER

Fax +41 61 306 12 34
E-Mail karger@karger.ch
www.karger.com

1021–7401/10/0173–0161$26.00/0

Accessible online at:
www.karger.com/nim

Elena Gonzalez-Rey
Instituto de Parasitología y Biomedicina López-Neyra, CSIC
Avda. Conocimiento, PT Ciencias de la Salud
ES–18100 Granada (Spain)
Tel. +34 958 181 670, Fax +34 958 181 632, E-Mail elenag@ipb.csic.es

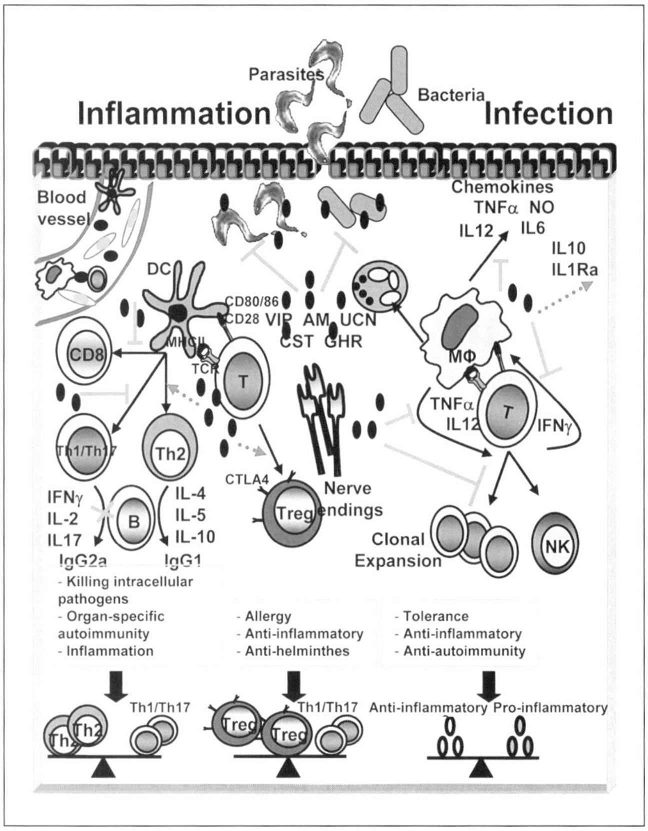

Fig. 1. Tuning the immune system with endogenous neuropeptides. Vasoactive intestinal peptide (VIP), adrenomedullin (AM), urocortin (UCN), cortistatin (CST), and ghrelin (GHR) are released from nerve terminals (nervous source) and blood (endocrine source), or produced by T helper 2 (TH2) cells or macrophages (immune source) in response to antigenic and inflammatory stimulation. Together with the recently discovered bactericidal and trypanolytic effect, these neuropeptides have an immunomodulatory role exerted by different nonexcluding mechanisms. First, they induce the generation and differentiation of TH2 cell functions and decrease TH1 cell responses. As a consequence, the inflammatory and autoimmune responses are impaired. Second, these peptides inhibit the production of inflammatory cytokines, chemokines and free radicals by macrophages. In addition, they impair the costimulatory activity of APCs on effector T cells, inhibiting subsequent clonal expansion. This avoids the inflammatory response and its cytotoxic effect against the target tissue. Third, they induce the generation of regulatory T cells that suppress the activation of autoreactive T cells. All these mechanisms contribute to the maintenance of an anti-inflammatory state, avoid undesired immunopathologies resulting from infection, and restores immune tolerance. Dashed lines indicate positive stimulation. End-braked lines represent inhibition. CTLA4 = Cytotoxic T lymphocyte-associated protein 4; TCR = T cell receptor; TNF-α = tumor-necrosis factor-α; Treg = regulatory T cell.

it is important to consider that there is not a solely immune response, but some factors produced by the neuroendocrine system could also contribute to the maintenance of immune tolerance. For example, glucocorticoids and noradrenaline, endogenous immunosuppressive agents, are produced by the HPA axis and the sympathetic nervous system, respectively, in response to stress or systemic inflammation [1]. Neuropeptides are also released by sensory and efferent nerves in close proximity to immune cells, in response to various invasive and inflammatory stimuli.

Here, we focus on some newly discovered anti-inflammatory neuropeptides, which keep the communication between the neuroendocrine and immune systems able to participate in the homeostasis of the organisms. Vasoactive intestinal peptide (VIP), urocortin (UCN), adrenomedullin (AM), cortistatin (CST) and ghrelin (GHR) belong to different families of peptides, with no homology between them. They have different cellular sources, physiological roles in the body and receptors. However, these neuropeptides have common characteristics that make them attractive from a point of view of maintenance of immune tolerance: all of them are produced by immune cells, especially under inflammatory conditions or following antigenic stimulation; they bind to G-protein-coupled receptors (GPCRs) expressed in different immunocompetent cells, and they mainly signal through the activation of the cAMP-protein kinase A (PKA) pathway (an immunosuppressive signal).

We have studied the immune role of these peptides. We have described that they modulate immune responses deactivating the inflammatory responses, inhibiting autoreactive populations and inducing tolerance (fig. 1). Treatment with VIP, UCN, AM, CST, or GHR decreases the frequency, delays the onset and reduces the severity of different established experimental models of sepsis, rheumatoid arthritis, inflammatory bowel disease, type 1 diabetes, and multiple sclerosis [2]. The therapeutic effect of these neuropeptides is associated with a striking reduction of a wide spectrum of inflammatory mediators as cytokines, chemokines, and free radicals involved in local and systemic damage. At the same time, they stimulate the production of anti-inflammatory cytokines such as IL-10 by macrophages, microglia and dendritic cells (DCs) (fig. 1). By contrast, neuropeptides reduce the autoreactive TH1 cell response and the subsequent titre of autoantibodies (particularly TH1-type IgG2a). Finally, these neuropeptides induce the peripheral expansion of new antigen-specific $CD4^+CD25^+$ fork head box P3 $(FOXP3)^+$ T regulatory cells [3]. Their suppressive activity on autoreactive T cells mechanism is mediated through direct cellular contact, which is mainly dependent on the production of cytotoxic T lymphocyte-associated protein 4 (CTLA4) or immunosuppressive cytokines IL-10 and/or TGF-b 1 (fig. 1). In addition, VIP generates DCs with a tolerogenic phenotype, characterized by their ability to induce CD4 and CD8 regulatory T cells [4]. The generation of regulatory T cells has recently been found to have a major role in the beneficial effect of these neuropeptides in autoimmunity.

Regarding the main actions of these peptides in the immune system, we could think that they deactivate the immune response and therefore they could cause some kind of immunosuppression and influence the natural response against infection. Contrary to the expected results, septic mice treated with these peptides had lower peritoneal bacterial counts than untreated mice [5]. Interestingly, we and others have shown that some of these neuropeptides such as AM and GHR are able to exert a direct antibacterial effect. In fact, these neuropeptides resemble antimicrobial peptides sharing with them some properties: (1) neuropeptides are found in primitive organisms and are highly conserved; (2) they are inducible under inflammation, produced by epithelial and mucosal surfaces, and (3) they are small peptides with high positive charge and amphipathic design. In general, antimicrobial peptides target and destroy the negatively charged membranes of pathogens, including bacteria, viruses, fungi, or parasites. Our results suggest that neuropeptides affect the bacteria viability by disrupting the integrity of the cell membrane [5].

Although some antimicrobial peptides have been successfully used against pathogens, their potential role against parasites is mostly unknown. In this sense, some cationic antimicrobial peptides such as cecropin and mellitin (of insect origin) or defensins and cathelicidins (produced by leukocytes and epithelial cells) kill protozoan parasites by disrupting plasma membrane integrity and leading to osmotic instability and lysis. Their mechanism of action is based on the fact that these trypanosomatids also have a highly negative charged coat. These parasites produce some of the neglected tropical diseases, and affect almost 500 million people over the world. The current treatment is antiquated, ineffective, toxic, and susceptible to resistance by the parasite. This has generated the urgent need of developing new therapeutic approaches that should include agents with nontraditional modes of action. We propose that the neuropeptides could exert a direct lethal effect against parasites, based on their antimicrobial properties. We showed that various endogenous peptides act as potent anti-trypanosome agents killing the bloodstream forms of *Trypanosoma brucei*, the causing agent of the sleeping sickness [6]. The trypanolytic activity of the neuropeptides against *T. brucei* is completely different from that described for antimicrobial peptides. It involves peptide uptake and accumulation into intracellular vesicles, disruption of lysosome integrity and cytosolic accumulation of glycolytic enzymes. This promotes an energetic metabolism failure that initiates an autophagic-like cell death [6]. In an animal model of chronic trypanosomiasis, neuropeptide-based treatment improved clinical signs. They decreased parasite burden in target tissues and significantly delayed death of infected mice. From a therapeutic point of view, targeting intracellular compartments by neuropeptides supposes a new promising strategy for the treatment of parasitic diseases that overcome resistances. Of physiological importance is the fact that the hosts respond to trypanosome infection producing neuropeptides as part of their natural innate defense.

Together, the immunomodulatory role of the neuropeptides and their action in response to the infectious process should provide insight into therapeutic approaches for the control of autoimmune/inflammatory and infectious diseases. As small and hydrophilic molecules, neuropeptides are attractive compounds for treating excessive inflammation because their permeability properties that enable rapid access to the site of inflammation. They have a wide and potent spectrum of action mainly due to their high-affinity binding to specific receptors. As for other drugs, we should consider the potential side effects as a consequence of the other effects of these neuropeptides in the body, such as hypotension, decreased gut motility, endocrine disorders, diarrhea, and disturbances in circadian rhythm and memory. It is important to note that some of these neuropeptides have already been tested in humans for the treatment of sepsis and other disorders [7–9], without such complications. Therefore, in contrast to existing anti-inflammatory drugs, neuropeptides are not associated with dramatic side effects because being physiological compounds, they are intrinsically nontoxic. Neuropeptides are rapidly cleared from the body through natural hepatic detoxification mechanisms and renal excretion. Moreover, other cytokines, neuropeptides and hormones often counterbalance their actions, and the homeostasis of normal tissues is not perturbed. Despite these advantages, several obstacles stand between translating neuropeptide-based treatment into viable clinical therapies. Due to their natural structural conformation, neuropeptides are highly unstable and extremely sensitive to peptidases present in most tissues. Several strategies have been developed to increase neuropeptide half-life, especially in long-term treatments. Pharmaceutical companies are trying the development of metabolically stable analogs. However, in the case of the type 2 GPCRs (i.e. receptors for VIP, urocortin, α-MSH and adrenomedullin), the pharmaceutical industry has so far failed to generate effective specific, non-peptide agonists [10]. Understanding of the structure-function relationship of these neuropeptides and their specific receptors, including receptor signaling, internalization, and homo- and heterodimerization, will facilitate the development of novel pharmacological agents. Meanwhile, we should focus on develop new strategies to allow the direct use of natural peptides. For example, modifications in the sequence or cycling the structure increase the stability of these peptides. Improving neuropeptide delivery to target tissues and cells while protecting them against degradation include strategies based on neuropeptide gene delivery, the insertion of VIP into micelles or nanoparticles, or combining neuropeptide treatment with inhibitors of endopeptidases. Alternatively, administration of serum-specific neuropeptide-binding proteins (e.g. AMBP-1) might protect them from peptidases and enhance their delivery in the proximity of their receptors in the inflamed tissue.

Collectively, the findings described here show the tremendous plasticity of these neuropeptides for the clinical translation to human immune and/or infectious disorders.

In fact, recent studies have shown the relevance of these neuropeptides to health as alterations in the endogenous levels of these agents and their receptors are associated with onset of certain autoimmune and inflammatory processes. These results suggest that a healthy neuropeptide network is necessary to upset the balance of body systems and get the homeostasis that allows survival.

References

1 Sternberg EM: Neural regulation of innate immunity: a coordinated nonspecific host response to pathogen. Nat Rev Immunol 2006;6:318–328.
2 Varela N, Chorny A, Gonzalez-Rey E, Delgado M: Tuning inflammation with anti-inflammatory neuropeptides. Expert Opin Biol Ther 2007;7:461–478.
3 Gonzalez-Rey E, Chorny A, Delgado M: Regulation of immune tolerance by anti-inflammatory neuropeptides Nat Rev Immunol 2007;7:52–63.
4 Chorny A, Gonzalez-Rey E, Fernandez-Martin A, Pozo D, Ganea D, Delgado M: Vasoactive intestinal peptide induces regulatory dendritic cells with therapeutic effects on autoimmune disorders. Proc Natl Acad Sci USA 2005;102:13562–13567.
5 Chorny A, Anderson P, Gonzalez-Rey E, Delgado M: Ghrelin protects against experimental sepsis by inhibiting high-mobility group box 1 release and by killing bacteria. J Immunol 2008;180:8369–8377.
6 Delgado M, Anderson P, Garcia-Salcedo JA, Caro M, Gonzalez-Rey E: Neuropeptides kill African trypanosomes by targeting intracellular compartments and inducing autophagic-like cell death. Cell Death Differ 2009;16: 406–416.
7 Nagaya N, Satoh T, Nishikimi T, Uematsu M, Furuichi S, Sakamaki F, Oya H, Kyotani S, Nakanishi N, Goto Y, Masuda Y, Miyatake K, Kangawa K: Hemodynamic, renal, and hormonal effects of adrenomedullin infusion in patients with congestive heart failure. Circulation 2000;101:498–503.
8 Davis ME, Pemberton CJ, Yandle TG, Lainchbury JG, Rademaker MT, Nicholls MG, Frampton CM, Richards AM: Effect of urocortin 1 infusion in humans with stable congestive cardiac failure. Clin Sci 2005;109: 381–388.
9 Petkov V, Mosgoeller W, Ziesche R, Raderer M, Stiebellehner L, Vonbank K, Funk GC, Hamilton G, Novotny C, Burian B, Block LH: Vasoactive intestinal peptide as a new drug for treatment of primary pulmonary hypertension. J Clin Invest 2003;111:1339–1346.
10 Blakeney JS, Fairlie DP: Nonpeptide ligands that target peptide-activated GPCRs in inflammation. Curr Med Chem 2005;12:3027–3042.

NeuroImmunoModulation

Neuroimmunomodulation 2010;17:165–168
DOI: 10.1159/000258714

Published online: February 4, 2010

When Immune-Neuro-Endocrine Interactions Are Disrupted: Experimentally Induced Arthritis as an Example

Adriana del Rey[a] Christine Wolff[b] Johannes Wildmann[a] Anke Randolf[a] Rainer H. Straub[b] Hugo O. Besedovsky[a]

[a]Department of Immunophysiology, Institute of Physiology and Pathophysiology, Medical Faculty, Marburg, and [b]Laboratory of Experimental Rheumatology and Neuroendocrino-Immunology, Department of Internal Medicine I, University Hospital Regensburg, Regensburg, Germany

Key Words

Arthritis · Hypothalamus-pituitary-adrenal axis · Sympathetic nervous system · Brain-borne cytokines · Neurotransmitters · Hypothalamus · Denervation

Abstract

We studied whether, in parallel to the activity of the hypothalamus-pituitary-adrenal axis and the sympathetic nervous system, hypothalamic cytokine expression and monoaminergic neurotransmitter concentrations are affected during the development and chronification of arthritis induced by immunization of rats with type II collagen. Corticosterone levels were increased only transiently, and were even below the normal range as the disease progressed. Increased adrenaline blood levels and hypothalamic IL-1β and IL-6 overexpression were observed only during the induction phase of the disease. The increase in hypothalamic noradrenaline content during the symptomatic phase was paralleled by a gradual loss of sympathetic fibers in the joints. Depletion of hypothalamic noradrenergic neurons at this time did not affect the symptomatology. Contrary to observations in healthy animals, no correlation between hypothalamic IL-1β expression and noradrenaline content was observed in rats with arthritis. The dissociation between hypothalamic cytokine gene expression and noradrenergic neuronal activity, the lack of sustained stimulation of the stress axes, and the loss of sympathetic signals in the joints indicate that the communication between afferent immune messages to the central nervous system and two main efferent anti-inflammatory pathways under control of the brain are disrupted during experimental arthritis.

Rheumatoid arthritis (RA) is a peripheral polyarthritis of unknown etiology (for review, see [1]). The disease is characterized by synovitis, joint swelling, tenderness, destruction and pain, morning stiffness and limitation of joint mobility. If untreated, the joint inflammation results in cartilage and bone erosion, leading to joint deformity and damage with the consequent loss of function. It can spread to other joints within months to years, ending in disability, which can be very severe. Genetic factors, such as certain HLA-DR alleles and non-MHC (major histocompatibility complex) genes (e.g. PTNP 22) account for about 50% of the risk of developing RA. Environmental factors, for example infection with certain agents, among which are Epstein-Barr virus, *Mycobacterium tuberculosis*, *Escherichia coli*, and *Parvovirus*, have

KARGER

Fax +41 61 306 12 34
E-Mail karger@karger.ch
www.karger.com

1021–7401/10/0173–0165$26.00/0

Accessible online at:
www.karger.com/nim

Adriana del Rey
Department of Immunophysiology, Institute of Physiology and Pathophysiology
Medical Faculty, Deutschhausstrasse 2
DE–35037 Marburg (Germany)
Tel. +49 6421 286 2175, Fax +49 6421 286 8925, E-Mail delrey@mailer.uni-marburg.de

been proposed as a contributing cause to the development of the disease, but no consistent associations have been demonstrated. Autoimmune processes are undoubtedly involved in the pathogenesis of RA. This is clearly evidenced by its MHC dependence, indicating T cell involvement in the process, and by the production of autoantibodies. Rheumatoid factor (RF) is detected in approximately 80% of the RA patients, and the titers correlate with the severity of the disease. Antibodies against cyclic-citrullinated peptides (CCP) are highly specific for RA. RF and anti-CCP considered together are present in more than 90% of the patients.

Activated T cells, macrophages and plasma cells are found in the synovial membrane of the compromised joints. Neutrophils in the synovial fluid, together with changes in other parameters, such as increased expression of Toll-like receptors in the synovium, indicate that the innate immune system is also activated during RA. An explanation for the development of this disease based on the 'classical' Th1-Th2 paradigm is now considered too simplistic. At present, the balance between Th17 and T regulatory (Treg) cells seems to be more important, as indicated by the finding that Tregs from RA patients fail to suppress cytokine production by T cells and monocytes. There is a lot of evidence that pro- and anti-inflammatory cytokines play a pivotal role within the affected joint. Particularly TNF-α and IL-1β are involved in the inflammatory and destructive processes of RA. TNF-α mediates pathologic inflammation, joint destruction, and systemic, extra-articular, inflammatory symptoms, and regulates the levels of adhesion molecules responsible for leukocyte migration. IL-1 also actively participates in the pathological process. It activates monocytes and macrophages, leading to inflammation; induces fibroblast proliferation, which results in the formation of a synovial pannus, and activates chrondrocytes, causing cartilage breakdown, and osteoclasts, an effect that contributes to bone resorption (for review, see [1]).

As with most chronic diseases, why the pathological process is not controlled and why it does not resolve remain open key questions also in RA. Our approach to this problem consisted in studying whether alterations in immune-neuro-endocrine interactions might also be involved in RA pathology [2]. For this purpose, we used an animal model in which arthritis was induced in DA rats by inoculation of bovine type II collagen (CII) suspended in incomplete Freund's adjuvant (IFA). Three groups of rats that received either saline solution (0.9% NaCl), or CII alone, or IFA only, served as controls. Several neuroendocrine parameters and cytokine production were evaluated in parallel to the development of the typical symptomatology. There are several procedures to induce arthritis experimentally that mainly differ in the way of inducing the disease and the rat strain used. Thus, we first evaluated parameters that could indicate whether eventual alterations in immune-neuro-endocrine interactions might be extrapolated to the human disease, albeit the limitations of any animal model.

All parameters were determined in parallel in the same rats. The first symptoms of disease, as scored by signs of inflammation in the affected joints, appeared around 14 days after CII+IFA injection, reached a maximum around day 28, and were maintained at this level in all immunized rats until the end of the studies, on day 55. None of the animals in the other three groups developed any clinical symptom. As expected, lymphoid cells obtained from the draining lymph nodes of CII+IFA-injected rats and cultured in vitro without further stimulation produced increasing amounts of TNF-α and IFN-γ as the disease progressed; increased IL-1β production was detected only until day 14, and IL-10 secretion was markedly increased during the chronic phase.

Markedly increased corticosterone blood levels were detected only on day 5 after immunization, but the levels decreased with the progression of the disease, and were even below those of the control rats towards the end of the studies. Increased adrenaline plasma levels were also detected on day 5 and the levels were maintained elevated at least until day 28 after immunization. The quantification of nerve fibers containing tyrosine hydroxylase (the rate-limiting enzyme in noradrenaline synthesis) in the joints of the arthritic rats showed that the sympathetic innervation gradually disappears as the disease progresses, and significant differences were observed already 28 days after immunization. Thus, similar to the disease in RA patients [3–5], relatively low glucocorticoid levels during the chronic phase, hyperactivity of the sympathetic nervous system (SNS), and reduction of sympathetic nerve fibers in the inflamed joints were also observed in arthritic rats.

The next set of determinations was performed in the hypothalamus of the four groups of rats, evaluations that obviously cannot be done in RA patients. The concentrations of serotonin and its main metabolite 5-HIAA were increased, resp. decreased, in the hypothalamus of arthritic rats at the last time point studied. The most sustained change in hypothalamic neurotransmitters was a marked increase in NA concentration, which was significant already 28 days after immunization and was main-

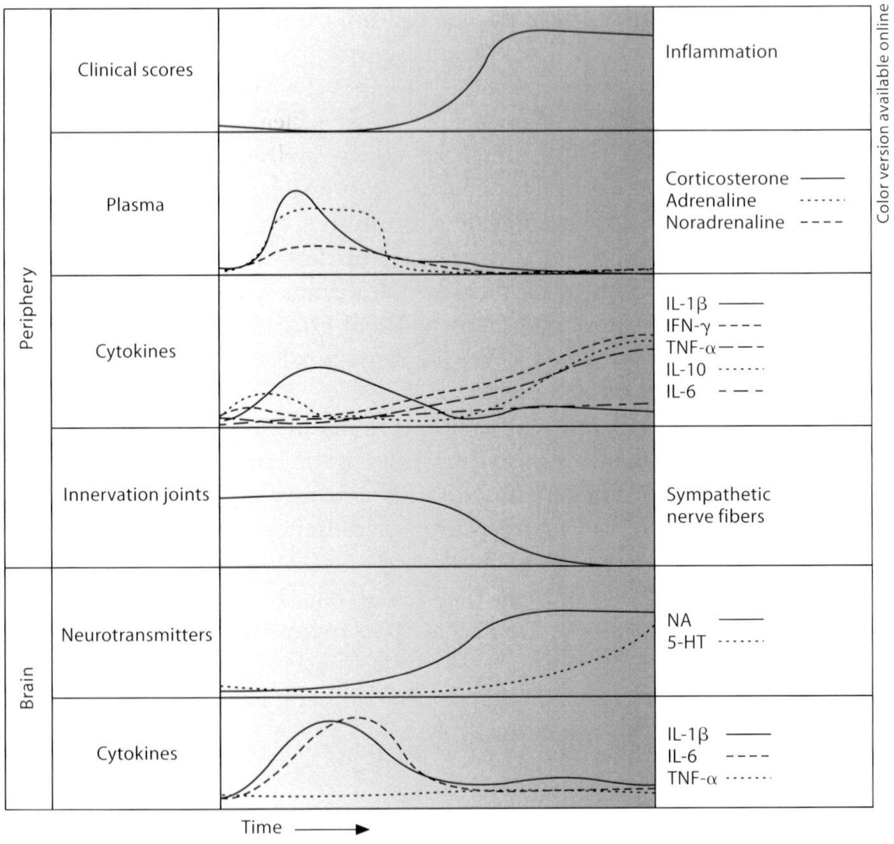

Fig. 1. Schematic representation of changes in peripheral and central parameters during the development and progression of experimentally induced arthritis. The different temporal responses of the HPA and the sympathetic nervous system, central and peripheral cytokine production, and hypothalamic cytokine expression and neurotransmitter content can be appreciated.

tained increased until the end of the studies. Contrary to our expectation, IL-1β and IL-6 (but not TNF-α) genes were significantly overexpressed in the hypothalamus of arthritic rats only during the induction phase. These results are schematically represented in figure 1. Interestingly, while there was a positive correlation between NA concentration and IL-1 gene expression in the hypothalamus of the three control groups, this correlation was not apparent in arthritic rats.

Finally, as an attempt to study the relevance of the increased NA concentration during disease development, noradrenergic neurons in the brain of arthritic rats were depleted by i.c.v. injection of the neurotoxin 6-hydroxydopamine when animals already showed clear clinical symptoms of arthritis. This treatment did not affect the clinical score.

Taken together, the results described indicate that brain-integrated neuro-endocrine responses are disorganized and disrupted during the inflammatory/immune response that causes arthritis, even before symptoms of the disease are detected. The arguments that support this proposal are as follows.

(1) It is very well established that pro-inflammatory cytokines can stimulate the hypothalamus-pituitary-adrenal (HPA) axis (for review, see [6]). Thus, the progressive decrease in corticosterone blood levels during the chronic phase of arthritis, when the production of cytokines that can stimulate the HPA axis is markedly increased in the periphery, indicates a disruption between the HPA axis and the immune system.
(2) Stimulation of the HPA axis and the SNS usually occurs in parallel, as it happens, for example, during a stress response. During arthritis, however, the increase in blood adrenaline is much more prolonged than the activation of the HPA axis, suggesting an uncoupling of the stress axes.
(3) It is well established that the SNS mediates immunoregulatory signals (for review, see [7]). The spontaneous sympathetic denervation of the joints during RA impedes the transmission of these modulatory effects.
(4) IL-1β is one of the most potent cytokines to stimulate the HPA axis (for review, see [6]). However, an increased IL-1β expression in the hypothalamus during

the induction phase of the disease did not result in stimulation of this axis. These results suggest that interactions between brain-borne IL-1 and the HPA axis are missing in this pathology.

(5) Several groups, including ours, have shown that peripheral cytokines can induce cytokine expression in the brain, and that glucocorticoids can inhibit cytokine production. However, no increase in pro-inflammatory cytokine expression in the hypothalamus was observed during the symptomatic phase of arthritis, when peripheral cytokine production is maximal and there is no activation of the HPA axis.

(6) Increased hypothalamic NA concentrations during arthritis are not paralleled by stimulation of the HPA axis, as it should be expected, indicating a disruption in the communication between central noradrenergic neurons and this axis.

(7) The positive correlation between hypothalamic IL-1β gene expression and NA content that exists in healthy animals is not observed in arthritic rats, suggesting that interactions between neural mechanisms and IL-1β are not functioning appropriately.

(8) We have previously shown that depletion of brain NA results in decreased peripheral immune responses, but that, when this treatment is combined with sympathectomy, such inhibition is lost [8]. These results agree with our observation that central NA depletion when the disease was well established and sympathetic innervation was lost spontaneously did not affect symptomatology.

In conclusion, taken together, the results support the proposal that multidirectional brain-immune system-joint interactions between cytokines conveying afferent signals to the central nervous system, brain-borne cytokines and neurotransmitters, and two main efferent neuro-endocrine anti-inflammatory pathways mediated by glucocorticoids and the SNS, become progressively disrupted during CII-induced arthritis.

Acknowledgement

This work was supported by the DFG (DE 1451/4-2).

References

1 Imboden JB: The immunopathogenesis of rheumatoid arthritis. Annu Rev Pathol 2009; 4:417–434.
2 del Rey A, Wolff C, Wildmann J, Randolf A, Hahnel A, Besedovsky HO, Straub RH: Disrupted brain-immune system-joint communication during experimental arthritis. Arthritis Rheum 2008;58:3090–3099.
3 Straub RH, Paimela L, Peltomaa R, Scholmerich J, Leirisalo-Repo M: Inadequately low serum levels of steroid hormones in relation to interleukin-6 and tumor necrosis factor in untreated patients with early rheumatoid arthritis and reactive arthritis. Arthritis Rheum 2002;46:654–662.
4 Bijlsma JW, Cutolo M, Straub RH, Masi AT: Clinical aspects of immune neuroendocrine mechanisms in rheumatic diseases. Rheum Dis Clin North Am 2005;31:xiii–xvii.
5 Weidler C, Holzer C, Harbuz M, Hofbauer R, Angele P, Scholmerich J, Straub RH: Low density of sympathetic nerve fibres and increased density of brain derived neurotrophic factor positive cells in RA synovium. Ann Rheum Dis 2005;64:13–20.
6 Besedovsky HO, del Rey A: Physiology of psychoneuroimmunology: a personal view. Brain Behav Immun 2007;21:34–44.
7 Elenkov IJ, Wilder RL, Chrousos GP, Vizi ES: The sympathetic nerve-an integrative interface between two supersystems: the brain and the immune system. Pharmacol Rev 2000;52:595–638.
8 Pacheco-Lopez G, Niemi MB, Kou W, Bildhauser A, Gross CM, Goebel MU, del Rey A, Besedovsky HO, Schedlowski M: Central catecholamine depletion inhibits peripheral lymphocyte responsiveness in spleen and blood. J Neurochem 2003;86:1024–1031.

NeuroImmunoModulation

Neuroimmunomodulation 2010;17:169–172
DOI: 10.1159/000258715

Published online: February 4, 2010

Effects of Stress on the Immune Response to Theiler's Virus – Implications for Virus-Induced Autoimmunity

C. Jane Welsh[a, b] Andrew J. Steelman[a] Wentao Mi[a] Colin R. Young[a]
Dana D. Dean[a] Ralph Storts[b] Thomas H. Welsh, Jr.[c] Mary W. Meagher[d]

Departments of [a]Veterinary Integrative Biosciences and [b]Veterinary Pathobiology, College of Veterinary Medicine and Biomedical Sciences, [c]Department of Animal Science, College of Agriculture and Life Sciences, and [d]Department of Psychology, College of Liberal Arts, Texas A&M University, College Station, Tex., USA

Key Words
Multiple sclerosis · Theiler's virus · Restraint stress · Innate immunity · Adaptive immunity

Abstract
Psychological stress is an important factor in susceptibility to many diseases. Our laboratory has been investigating the impact of stress on the susceptibility to Theiler's virus-induced demyelination (TVID), a mouse model of multiple sclerosis. Using immunodominant viral peptides specific for identification of either $CD4^+$ or $CD8^+$ T cells, stress reduced IFN-γ-producing virus-specific $CD4^+$ and $CD8^+$ T cells in the spleen and $CD8^+$ T cells in the CNS. Expression of mRNA for the Th1 transcription factor T-bet and the Th2 transcription factor GATA-3 were decreased in spleen cells isolated from stressed mice. Cytokine production by cells isolated from the CNS or spleens following stimulation with virus indicated that stress decreased both type 1 and type 2 responses. The adverse effects of stress were partially reversed by concurrent RU486 administration but mimicked by dexamethasone, indicating a major role for glucocorticoids. Global stress-induced immunosuppression resulted in higher levels of virus replication and dissemination. The higher viral load subsequently led to an earlier disease onset and more severe clinical and histological signs of demyelinating disease. Our results have important implications for understanding the pathogenesis of MS, and suggest that stressful events during early infection with an agent capable of inducing demyelination may result in immunosuppression and failure to eliminate the pathogen, which in turn may lead to the development of MS.

Stress and Multiple Sclerosis

Multiple sclerosis (MS) is the most common demyelinating disease of the central nervous system (CNS) affecting approximately 350,000 people in the US. The etiology of this disease is unknown, although viral infection during early adulthood is suspected as an initiating event followed by autoimmune-mediated demyelination. In common with other autoimmune diseases, stressful life events precipitate both the onset and clinical relapses in MS patients. One of the mechanisms by which stress affects MS is to compromise the immune system and lead to increased susceptibility to infections,

KARGER
Fax +41 61 306 12 34
E-Mail karger@karger.ch
www.karger.com

1021–7401/10/0173–0169$26.00/0

Accessible online at:
www.karger.com/nim

Dr. C. Jane Welsh
Department of Veterinary Integrative Biosciences
College of Veterinary Medicine and Biomedical Sciences
Texas A&M University, College Station, TX 77843-4458 (USA)
Tel. +1 979 862 4974, Fax +1 979 847 8981, E-Mail jwelsh@cvm.tamu.edu

which may contribute to MS onset and also exacerbations in established MS.

Since the earliest descriptions of MS, stress has been considered a controversial, but significant factor in the onset and course of the disease. Anecdotal accounts suggest that life stress frequently triggers the development of MS symptoms. Psychological stress has been implicated in the onset of MS, and acute life stressors have been shown to be correlated with relapses in established MS. A meta-analysis of 14 papers concerning stress and MS concluded that there was 'a significantly increased risk of exacerbation associated with stressful life events' [1]. However, the mechanisms underlying the role of stress in MS are complex and difficult to investigate in patients.

A Viral Etiology for Multiple Sclerosis

The etiology of MS is unknown, although epidemiological studies have implicated an infective agent as a possible initiating factor. Epidemiological surveys have shown that an increased risk of developing MS was associated with late infection with mumps, measles and Epstein-Barr virus. Additionally, exacerbations of MS are frequently preceded by viral infections. Interestingly, several viral agents including measles, mumps, parainfluenza type I, coronavirus, Epstein-Barr and human herpes type 6 have been detected in the brains of MS patients. Thus, it is intriguing that the antiviral, IFN-β, has been reported to have a beneficial effect on relapsing/remitting MS. One mechanism of stress-induced exacerbation might be via increased glucocorticoid secretion resulting in immunosuppression and reactivation of latent viruses, such as herpes virus.

Viruses are known to cause demyelination in experimental animal models: measles virus in rats; canine distemper virus in dogs; visna virus in sheep; JHM mouse hepatitis virus, Semliki Forest virus and Theiler's virus in mice. Therefore, in order to understand the pathogenesis of MS it is appropriate to study an animal model of virus-induced demyelination such as Theiler's virus infection. Theiler's virus infection in mice represents not only an excellent model for the study of the pathogenesis of MS but also a model system for studying disease susceptibility factors, mechanisms of viral persistence within the CNS and mechanisms of virus-induced autoimmune disease.

Theiler's Virus-Induced Demyelination as a Model for Multiple Sclerosis

Theiler's murine encephalomyelitis virus is a Picornavirus that causes an asymptomatic gastrointestinal infection and occasionally paralysis in mice. Following intracerebral infection, susceptible strains of mice develop a primary inflammatory demyelination with similarities to MS. The immune system plays a crucial role in early clearance of viral infection from the CNS, via activation of NK cells, anti-viral $CD4^+$ and $CD8^+$ T cells and also through the generation of virus-specific antibodies. Susceptible mice fail to clear the virus from the CNS and consequently develop the late demyelinating disease. In the late disease, the immune system takes on a pathogenic role in demyelination and CNS destruction.

Effects of Restraint Stress on the Innate Immune Response to Theiler's Virus

Our group has been investigating the effect of stress on the pathogenesis of Theiler's virus-induced demyelination (TVID). Using the restraint stress model we have shown that chronic stress increased: glucocorticoid secretion, sickness behavior, viral titers in the CNS and mortality following infection with Theiler's murine encephalomyelitis virus [2]. Restraint stress also decreased innate immune function, in particular NK cell activity [3], chemokine [4] and cytokine expression in the spleen and CNS [5] which resulted in decreased inflammatory cell infiltrates into the CNS [6].

Effects of Restraint Stress on the Adaptive Immune Response to Theiler's Virus

Furthering these studies, we have also shown that restraint stress reduces the adaptive immune response to Theiler's virus. In these experiments, mice were assigned to treatment groups and (1) either stressed overnight commencing day-1 and infected at day 0 and then stressed each night for 8 nights; (2) stressed at day-1 and mock infected with sterile phosphate-buffered saline at day 0, and then stressed each night for 8 nights; (3) nonstressed and infected at day 0; (4) nonstressed and mock infected at day 0. Then at day 8 postinfection, specific T cell responses were measured in the spleen and CNS using virus-specific ELSIPOT assays. We observed that stress reduced splenic $CD4^+$ and $CD8^+$ T cell responses to virus, and sig-

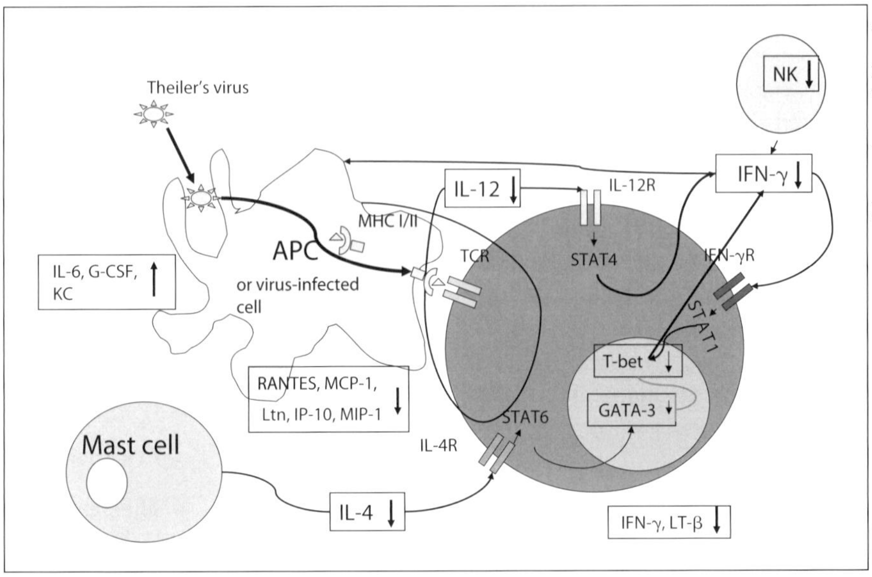

Color version available online

Fig. 1. The effects of stress on the immune response to Theiler's virus. Restraint stress induces increased production of glucocorticoids which cause global immunosuppression in Theiler's virus-infected mice. Stress-induced effects are contained within boxes: decreases are denoted by a downward arrow and increases by an upward arrow. Theiler's virus is taken up either by antigen-presenting cells such as macrophages or dendritic cells or infects other cell types. Antigen processing occurs and viral peptides are presented to T cells via their T cell receptor (TCR) in the context of the major histocompatibility complex (MHC I/II). Natural killer cell activity is reduced by stress and also the production of IFN-γ is reduced, which in turn reduces the activation of macrophages and T cells through signal transducers and activators of transcription (STAT)1 signaling. Th1 cells are driven by the transcription factor T-bet and activated by IL-12 through STAT4-signaling pathways. Th2 T cell responses are driven by GATA-3 and activation by IL-4 secretion and STAT6 signaling. Stress reduces the amount of IL-12 secreted by the antigen-presenting cells and then reduces the activation state of the Th1 cells. Stress also reduces mRNA expression of both T-bet and GATA-3 and thereby reduces both Th1 and Th2 responses. Stress also decreases the production of Ltn, IP-10, RANTES, MIP-1 and MCP-1 which reduces the inflammatory cell infiltrate into the CNS. Stress also reduces the expression of LT-β which has anti-viral properties along with IFN-γ and this may also contribute to the increased viral titers seen in the CNS. Interestingly, stress increases IL-6, G-CSF and KC. The increased KC production may account for the increased numbers of circulating neutrophils.

nificant reductions were noted in the number of IFN-γ-producing CNS infiltrating antiviral $CD8^+$ T cells [7]. Stress also reduced the mRNA levels for the Th1 transcription factor T-bet and the Th2 transcription factor GATA3. In addition, virus-induced Th1 and Th2 cytokine levels were also decreased. This indicates that stress causes suppression in both Th1 and Th2 T cell responses rather than a Th1 to Th2 switch.

Glucocorticoids were implicated as the main mediators of the stress-induced immunosuppression seen in these experiments since we were able to partially reverse the effects by concurrent administration of the glucocorticoid/progesterone antagonist mifpristone (RU486), and conversely we were able to mimic the effects by administration of the synthetic glucocorticoid dexamethasone [7].

In earlier studies of chemokine expression in the CNS, we noted a stress-induced decrease in virally induced RANTES, Ltn, and IL-10 [4]. Stress decreased levels of circulating chemokines: RANTES and MCP-1 [7]. Interestingly, IL-6, G-CSF and KC were increased by stress. The stress-induced increase in both G-CSF, a neutrophil hematopoietic factor, and KC, a neutrophil chemoattractant may account for the increase in circulating neutrophils we have previously observed in stressed mice [2]. All these data are diagrammatically displayed in figure 1 which explains the effect of stress on the immune response to Theiler's virus.

Chronic Stress Exacerbates the Demyelinating Phase of TVID

Mice subjected to chronic restraint stress during the first 4 weeks of Theiler's virus infection developed more severe demyelinating disease during the late phase of the disease [8]. Taken together with our observations on the effects of stress on the immune response to Theiler's virus, we propose that stress induces high concentrations of glucocorticoids which results in immunosuppression, reduced ability to clear virus and subsequently increased inflammatory demyelinating disease. Additionally, restraint stress facilitated the systemic dissemination of Theiler's virus resulting in increased viral replication in the heart and the development of a cardiotropic variant of the virus that induced pathology in the heart [6].

The phenomena of stress-induced immunosuppression leading to increased viral replication in the CNS of Theiler's murine encephalomyelitis virus-infected mice was also observed in two more naturalistic stress models, social disruption stress [9] and maternal separation stress [10].

Conclusions

Our work has shown that stress has a global immunosuppressive effect on the immune response to Theiler's virus and that glucocorticoids play a key role in this phenomenon. Both Th1 and Th2 responses are decreased by stress as indicated by decreased transcription factors T-bet and GATA-3 and Th1/Th2 cytokine responses. The decreased immune response to Theiler's virus leads to increased viral titers in the CNS and also increased viral dissemination. Relating our findings to the impact of stress on humans, we propose that stress would make an individual more susceptible to viral infections that might lead to the development of autoimmune diseases such as MS or indirectly precipitate MS relapse.

Acknowledgments

This research was funded by grants to C.J.W. and M.W.M. from the National Multiple Sclerosis Society RG 3128 and NIH/NINDS R01 39569 and NIH/NINDS R01-NS060822 awarded to M.W.M. and C.J.W. A.J.S. received support from the Recovery of Function Graduate Training Program, NIH/NRSA 5T32AI052 'Mechanistic studies at the host-pathogen interface' and performed this work in partial fulfillment of the requirements for the PhD degree at Texas A&M University, College Station, Tex., USA.

References

1 Mohr DC, Hart SL, Julian L, Cox D, Pelletier D: Association between stressful life events and exacerbation in multiple sclerosis: a meta-analysis. Br Med J 2004;328:731–735.

2 Campbell T, Meagher MW, Sieve A, Scott B, Storts R, Welsh TH, Welsh CJR: The effects of restraint stress on the neuropathogenesis of Theiler's virus infection. I. Acute disease. Brain Behav Immun 2001;15:235–254.

3 Welsh CJR, Bustamante L, Nayak M, Welsh TH, Dean DD, Meagher MW: The effects of restraint stress on the neuropathogenesis of Theiler's virus infection II: NK cell function and cytokine levels in acute disease. Brain Behav Immun 2004;18:166–174.

4 Mi W, Belyavskyi M, Johnson RR, Sieve AN, Storts R, Meagher MW, Welsh CJR: Alterations in chemokine expression in Theiler's virus infection and restraint stress. Neuroimmunology 2004;151:103–115.

5 Sieve AN, Steelman AJ, Young CR, Storts R, Welsh TH, Welsh C Jr, Meagher MW: Chronic restraint stress during early Theiler's virus infection exacerbates the subsequent demyelinating disease in SJL mice. J Neuroimmunol 2004;155:103–118.

6 Johnson RR, Prentice T, Bridegam P, Young CR, Steelman AJ, Welsh TH, Welsh CJR, Meagher MW: Social stress alters the severity and onset of the chronic phase of Theiler's virus infection. J Neuroimmunol 2006;175:39–51.

7 Mi W, Young CR, Storts R, Steelman A, Meagher MW, Welsh CJR: Stress alters pathogenicity and facilitates systemic dissemination of Theiler's virus. Microb Pathogen 2006;41:133–143.

8 Mi W, Prentice TW, Young CR, Johnson RR, Sieve AN, Meagher MW, Welsh CJR: Restraint stress decreases virus-induced proinflammatory cytokine expression during acute Theiler's virus infection. J Neuroimmunol 2006;178:49–61.

9 Steelman AJ, Dean DD, Young CR, Smith R, Prentice TW, Meagher MW, Welsh CJR: Restraint stress modulates virus specific adaptive immunity during acute Theiler's virus infection. Brain Behav Immun 2009;23:830–843.

10 Meagher MW, Sieve AN, Johnson RR, Satterlee D, Belyavskyi M, Mi W, Prentice TW, Welsh TH, Welsh CJR: Neonatal maternal separation alters immune, endocrine, and behavioral responses to acute Theiler's virus infection in adult mice. Behav Genet 2009;in press.

NeuroImmunoModulation

Neuroimmunomodulation 2010;17:173–176
DOI: 10.1159/000258716

Published online: February 4, 2010

Disease-Modifying Immunotherapy for the Management of Autoimmune Diabetes

Carla N. Castro[a] Andres E. Barcala Tabarrozi[a] Maria Antunica Noguerol[a] Ana C. Liberman[a] Ricardo A. Dewey[b] Eduardo Arzt[a] Adrian E. Morelli[c] Marcelo J. Perone[a]

[a]Laboratorio de Fisiología y Biología Molecular (LFBM)-IFIBYNE-CONICET, Facultad de Ciencias Exactas y Naturales, Universidad de Buenos Aires, Buenos Aires, and [b]Laboratorio de Terapia Génica y Células Madre, Instituto de Investigaciones Biotecnológicas-Instituto Tecnológico de Chascomús (IIB-INTECH), CONICET-UNSAM, Chascomús, Argentina; [c]Department of Surgery and Immunology, Thomas E. Starzl Transplantation Institute, University of Pittsburgh Medical Center, Pittsburgh, Pa., USA

Key Words
Type 1 diabetes · Immunoregulation · Dendritic cells

Abstract
Type 1 diabetes (T1D) is a T cell-mediated autoimmune disease that destroys the insulin-secreting β-cells of the pancreas. It is now possible to predict those candidates that will progress to T1D before the full onset of the disease. Prevention of uncontrollable autoimmunity against β-cells in therapies for T1D is mandatory to preserve the β-cell mass. Therefore, immunomodulatory strategies directed to inhibiting the activity of self-reactive T cell clones as well as induction of regulatory T cells would be beneficial for prevention of T1D or recurrence of β-cell autoimmunity against islet cell allografts.

Insulin-dependent diabetes mellitus, or type 1 diabetes (T1D) is an autoimmune disease with an increasing incidence worldwide [1]. T1D is a multifactorial disorder in which both genetic and environmental factors confer susceptibility to the disease. The clinical manifestations of long-lasting hyperglycemia due to lack of endogenous insulin lead to vascular damage subsequently associated with kidney failure, heart diseases, retinopathy and neuropathy. Although clinical evidence has shown that insulin replacement ameliorates life-threatening complications of diabetes, its use is considered by no means a cure but a palliative, and it cannot prevent, at long term, disease-related complications in most patients.

Gene inheritance is associated with susceptibility and progression of T1D in humans and in murine models of natural disease development, e.g. the nonobese diabetic (NOD) mice. However, gene-predisposing factors are necessary but not sufficient determinants for T1D onset. Unknown environmental factors play an important role in progression of autoimmune disorders, and it is believed that they may also account for the current increment on the incidence of T1D [2]. Thus, the interplay be-

KARGER

Fax +41 61 306 12 34
E-Mail karger@karger.ch
www.karger.com

1021–7401/10/0173–0173$26.00/0

Accessible online at:
www.karger.com/nim

Marcelo J. Perone, PhD
Laboratorio de Fisiología y Biología Molecular, IFIBYNE-CONICET
Facultad de Ciencias Exactas y Naturales, Universidad de Buenos Aires
Ciudad Universitaria-Pabellón II-2° piso, Buenos Aires 1428 (Argentina)
Tel. +54 11 4576 3368, Fax +54 11 4576 3321, E-Mail mperone@fbmc.fcen.uba.ar

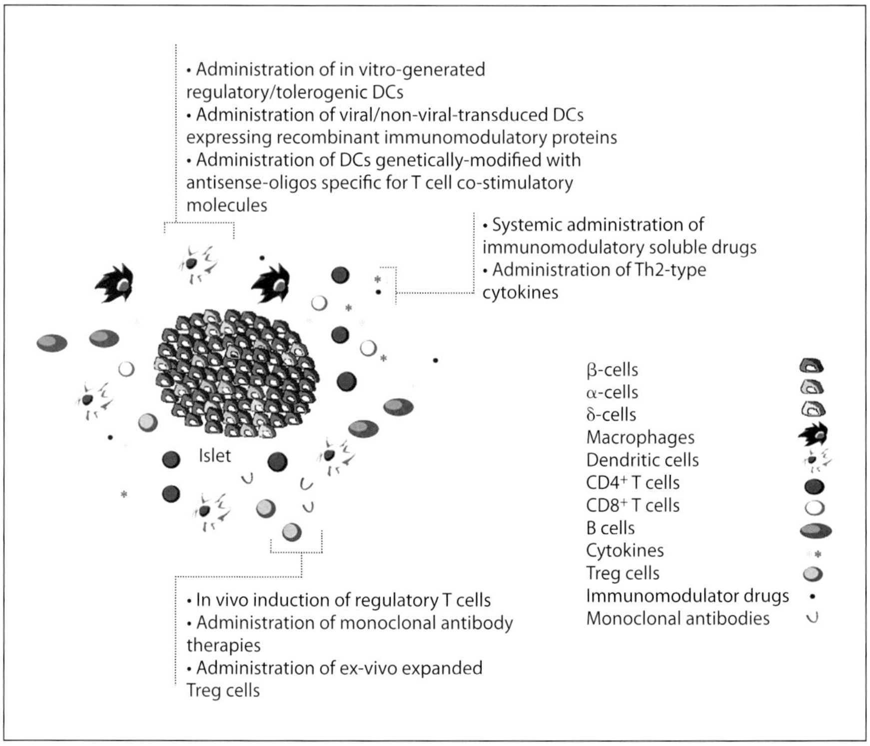

Color version available online

Fig. 1. Schematic diagram showing immune cells and cytokines involved in insulin-secreting β-cell specific autoimmune destruction during the T1D process. Putative therapeutic interventions are depicted targeting components of the immune system at different levels in order to re-establish a healthy balance.

tween gene susceptibility and environmental factors seems to be a key element triggering the autoimmune response and progression of diabetes, like in many other autoimmune disorders.

It is well known that T1D is a spontaneously developed T cell-mediated autoimmune disease that destroys the insulin-secreting β-cells of the islets of Langerhans in the pancreas. Accumulating evidence suggests that T1D occurs as a result of a chronic and progressive self-destruction of insulin-secreting β-cells. During the pathogenesis of the disease in NOD mice, the islets are firstly infiltrated by inflammatory leukocytes, mainly macrophages and dendritic cells (DCs), followed by T ($CD4^+$ and $CD8^+$) and B cells. In humans, there is accumulating evidence that a similar process takes place although with less degree of leukocyte infiltration of the islets [3].

The events that initiate T1D have not been fully elucidated. Agents of diverse nature have been associated to disregulation/disruption of the state of self-tolerance against β-cells. These agents may facilitate development of islet-specific T helper type 1 (Th1) clones, subsequently generating an imbalance of the Th1/Th2 ratio towards a prevalence to Th cells secreting type 1 cytokines, e.g. IFN-γ, TNF-α and IL-2.

Compelling evidence highlights the importance of $CD4^+$ T cells in the development and progression of T1D, such as the seminal observations that adoptive transference of diabetogenic $CD4^+$ T cells elicits autoimmune diabetes in young NOD mice and NOD*scid* mice [4]. Both, Th1 cell differentiation and the cytokine milieu present in and around the islets are thought to be critical for the development of T1D. It has been reported that Th1 cells and type 1 cytokines promote T1D in NOD mice whereas Th2 cells ameliorate/suppress the disease under certain experimental conditions. In fact, there is evidence that administration of immunomodulatory drugs protects against progression of T1D by promoting a shift from a Th1 to a Th2 response [5, 6]. However, so far, there is no conclusive evidence showing that a Th2 shift in the cytokine pattern leads to disease protection. In this regard, some studies have indicated that the Th1/Th2 shift represents a consequence, instead of the cause, of suppression of Th1-based autoimmunity in T1D.

In the past 5 years, in addition to Th1 and Th2 lymphocytes, Th17 cells have been proven to participate in host defenses against infectious agents, inflammatory and autoimmune diseases including rheumatoid arthritis and experimental autoimmune encephalitis, and allergy.

Nevertheless, the role of Th17 cells in autoimmune diabetes remains uncertain. Given that naïve Th cells exposed to a TGF-β/IL-6-rich microenvironment, cytokines frequently present in inflammatory conditions, differentiate into Th17 cells, it is tempting to speculate that IL-17 could play a role in the initiation/maintenance of autoimmunity in T1D [7]. A recent study has demonstrated that in vitro-generated Th17 cells can be reprogrammed into other Th cell lineages. Interestingly, upon transfer of β-cell-specific Th17 cells into NOD*scid* mice, the Th cells lost their ability to produce IL-17 and differentiated into Th1 cells. However, Th17 cells remained stable after adoptive transfer in nonlymphopenic hosts [8]. The cytokine environment in which the inflammatory response takes place further influences the intrinsic plasticity showed by Th17 cells in lymphopenic hosts. Surprisingly, we did not find a substantial increment of IL-17 secretion and percentage of Th17 cells in splenocytes from diabetic or young nondiabetic NOD mice [6]. Despite these controversial findings on the role of IL-17 in T1D, a recent study has shown that inhibition of Th17 cells attenuates onset of spontaneous T1D in NOD mice [9]. In the same direction, administration of IL-25 (also known as IL-17E), a cytokine of the IL-17 family that inhibits Th17 cells and promotes Th2 responses, reversed onset of T1D and delayed recurrent β-cell autoimmunity after islet transplantation in a syngeneic model [9].

Since T1D is an autoimmune disorder and β-cell-specific T cells are determinants for disease onset and progression, therapies directed to counter-regulate at multiple levels the immune burden would be beneficial for treatment of autoimmune diabetes (fig. 1). Several strategies have been tested in experimental models, preclinical models and clinical trials, including induction of β-cell-specific regulatory T cells (Treg) and antilymphocyte monoclonal antibody therapies [10]. However, a permanent tolerance state against β-cell antigens without the undesirable side effects of general immune suppression has not been achieved so far. This suggests that new intervention therapies combining inhibitory antibodies and immunoregulatory agents are warranted. Also, drugs of diverse chemical nature have been employed successfully as prophylactic intervention in animal models of T1D, without apparent toxic effects [5].

Dendritic cells (DCs) are pivotal components of the immune system due to their unique role in the induction and modulation of T, B, and natural killer cell-driven responses. They are crucial antigen-presenting cells involved in T cell immunity and tolerance. In vitro-generated DCs can be further manipulated pharmacologically or genetically and acquire a regulatory/tolerogenic function. Given the central role of DCs in peripheral T cell tolerance, they constitute a potential therapeutic approach for therapy of dysregulated immune responses against self-antigens.

With the aim to be used as therapeutics, in vitro-generated regulatory/tolerogenic DCs have been systemically administered into NOD mice to suppress autoimmune diabetes by reducing the β-cell-specific Th1/Th2 balance and/or generation of Treg. The mechanisms through which anti-inflammatory and immunosuppressive agents generate regulatory/tolerogenic DCs are diverse and include the use of corticosteroids, eicosanoids/lipids, growth factors, sphingolipids, cytokines, etc. Also, genetically engineered DCs may be obtained by transducing DCs with recombinant viral vectors encoding immunoregulatory proteins. Galectin-1, an endogenous mammalian lectin with multiple immune-regulatory functions, has been shown to modulate DCs activity when expressed as a transgene [11]. Interestingly, administration of DCs expressing transgenic galectin-1 delayed onset of autoimmune diabetes in an adoptive transfer model of diabetes in NOD mice [12]. Treatment of prediabetic NOD mice with DCs pre-incubated with anti-sense oligonucleotides of T cell costimulatory molecules prevented T1D onset by inducing Treg and Th2 cells [13].

In most autoimmune diseases like T1D, signs/symptoms that lead to diagnosis are mainly detected after the onset of the disease, when self-reactive T cells are already fully activated. Strategies targeting key cell components of the immune system very early in the progression of the disease could have potential clinical application, because they would allow for the preservation of the residual β-cell mass.

References

1 Atkinson MA, Eisenbarth GS: Type1 diabetes: new perspectives on disease pathogenesis and treatment. Lancet 2001;358:221–229.

2 Bach JF: The effect of infections on susceptibility to autoimmune and allergic diseases. N Engl J Med 2002;347:911–920.

3 Willcox A, Richardson SJ, Bone AJ, Foulis AK, Morgan NG: Analysis of islet inflammation in human type 1 diabetes. Clin Exp Immunol 2008;155:173–181.

4 Christianson SW, Shultz LD, Leiter EH: Adoptive transfer of diabetes into immunodeficient NOD-SCID/SCID mice: relative contributions of $CD4^+$ and $CD8^+$ T-cells from diabetic versus prediabetic NOD. NON-Thy-1a donors. Diabetes 1993;42:44–55.

5 Chang CLT, Chang SL, Lee YM, Chiang YM, Chuang DY, Kuo HK, Yang WC: Cytopiloyne, a polyacetylenic glucoside, prevents type 1 diabetes in nonobese diabetic mice. J Immunol 2007;178:6984–6993.
6 Perone MJ, Bertera S, Shufesky WJ, Divito SJ, Montecalvo A, Mathers AR, Larregina AT, Pang M, Seth N, Wucherpfennig KW, Trucco M, Baum LG, Morelli AE: Suppression of autoimmune diabetes by soluble galectin-1. J Immunol 2009;182:2641–2653.
7 Jain R, Tartar DM, Gregg RK, Divekar RD, Bell JJ, Lee H-H, Yu P, Ellis JS, Hoeman CM, Franklin CL, Zaghouani H: Innocuous IFNγ induced by adjuvant-free antigen restores normoglycemia in NOD mice through inhibition of IL-17 production. J Exp Med 2008; 205:207–218.
8 Nurieva R, Yang XO, Chung Y, Dong C: Cutting Edge: In vitro generated Th17 cells maintain their cytokine expression program in normal but not lymphopenic hosts. J Immunol 2009;182:2565–2568.
9 Emamaullee JA, Davis J, Merani S, Toso C, Elliott JF, Thiesen A, Shapiro AMJ: Inhibition of Th17 cells regulates autoimmune diabetes in NOD mice. Diabetes 2009;58:1302–1311.
10 Herold KC, Gitelman SE, Masharani U, Hagopian W, Bisikirska B, Donaldson D, Rother K, Diamond B, Harlan DM, Bluestone JA: A single course of anti-CD3 monoclonal antibody hOKT3{gamma}1(Ala-Ala) results in improvement in C-peptide responses and clinical parameters for at least 2 years after onset of type 1 diabetes. Diabetes 2005;54:1763–1769.
11 Perone MJ, Larregina AT, Shufesky WJ, Papworth GD, Sullivan MLG, Zahorchak AF, Stolz DB, Baum LG, Watkins SC, Thomson AW, Morelli AE: Transgenic galectin-1 induces maturation of dendritic cells that elicit contrasting responses on naïve and activated T cells. J Immunol 2006;176:7207–7220.
12 Perone MJ, Bertera S, Shufesky WJ, Zahorchak A, Piganelli J, Baum LG, Trucco M, Morelli AE: Dendritic cells expressing transgenic galectin-1 delay onset of autoimmune diabetes in mice. J Immunol 2006;177:5278–5289.
13 Machen J, Harnaha J, Lakomy R, Styche A, Trucco M, Giannoukakis N: Antisense oligonucleotides down-regulating costimulation confer diabetes-preventive properties to nonobese diabetic mouse dendritic cells. J Immunol 2004;173:4331–4341.

NeuroImmunoModulation

Neuroimmunomodulation 2010;17:177–179
DOI: 10.1159/000258717

Published online: February 4, 2010

Differential Regulation of IgG-NMO Autoantibodies on S100Beta Protein and Disability in Relapsing Neuromyelitis Optica

Maria A. Robinson-Agramonte[a] Carlos Alberto Saravia Gonçalves[b] Valmor L. Portela[b] A. Saiz-Hinarejos[c] Pierre J. Oses[b] Souza L. Motta[b] A. Pastoris Muller[b] M.E. Marquez Gonzalez[b] Onofre D. Gomes de Souza[b]

[a]International Center for Neurological Restoration and Cuban Neuroimmunology Society, Havana, Cuba; [b]Departamento de Bioquímica, Instituto de Ciências Básicas da Saúde, Universidade Federal do Rio Grande do Sul, Porto Alegre, Brazil; [c]Laboratory of Experimental Neurology and Immunology, Hospital Clinic Barcelona, Barcelona, Spain

Key Words

Neuromyelitis optica · Aquaporin 4 · Devic's disease · S-100beta · Glial cell markers · Demyelinating diseases

Abstract

Neuromyelitis optica (NMO), an uncommon central nervous system (CNS) demyelinating disease, produces transverse myelitis and severe optic neuritis. IgG-NMO autoantibody, a specific immunoglobulin binding aquaporin-4 water channel protein, confirms that NMO is a different entity to multiple sclerosis. Parallel to cytokine down-regulations found in serum of relapsing-NMO (rNMO) patients, it has been reported that IgG-NMO may also confer a worse course of the disease in r-NMO Caribbean patients. In this study, we were interested in exploring the influence of IgG-NMO autoantibody on S100β levels and clinical parameters from serum of r-NMO patients. Serum samples from 24 rNMO patients and 10 controls were evaluated. The reduction of S100β observed in r-NMO patients was not significant compared to controls; and no differences were present regarding IgG-NMO immunoreactivity. At the same time, a significant correlation was also observed between IgG-NMO autoantibody serum detection and EDSS (Expanded Disability Status Scale) in rNMO. These results corroborate a differential regulation of IgG-NMO autoantibodies on the S100β glial marker and on the disability present in rNMO patients.

Introduction

Neuromyelitis optica (NMO), a novel autoimmune type of channelopathy, is characterized by the co-occurrence of severe optic neuritis and longitudinal extensive transverse myelitis, either as monophasic or relapsing-remitting (rNMO) clinical forms [1]. Recently, a highly specific serum reactivity that targets aquaporin 4 (AQP4) in CNS microvessels, subpia and Virchow-Robin spaces (called IgG-NMO) has been found in about 78% of r-NMO patients from different populations [2].

As to the severity of the disease, research groups have attempted to identify lesional or disease activity markers in cerebrospinal fluid or serum of NMO patients, many of them comparing body fluid levels of markers between patients and controls [3, 4]. S100β is mainly localized to the glial cells and belongs to a family of calcium-binding proteins involved in intracellular and extracellular regu-

KARGER

Fax +41 61 306 12 34
E-Mail karger@karger.ch
www.karger.com

1021–7401/10/0173–0177$26.00/0

Accessible online at:
www.karger.com/nim

Maria A. Robinson-Agramonte
Department of Neuroimmunology, International Center for Neurological Restoration
Avenida 25 # 15805, e/n 158 y 160
Playa, Ciudad Habana 11300 (Cuba)
Tel. +53 7 271 6385, Fax +53 7 332 420, E-Mail maria.robinson@infomed.sld.cu

Table 1. S100β protein in serum of rNMO patients and control subjects

Groups	rNMO	rNMO (IgG^-NMO^+)	rNMO (IgG^-NMO^-)	Controls
Number	24	11	13	10
S100β, μg/ml	0.12 ± 0.016	0.11 ± 0.006	0.12 ± 0.021	0.16 ± 0.024

Groups studied were all rNMO patients (rNMO) and among them those positive (IgG^-NMO^+) or negative (IgG^-NOM^-) for autoantibodies.

latory activities like regulatory effects on cell growth, stimulation of neuronal survival, inhibition of the activity of inflammatory cells and neuronal death via apoptosis [5].

Besides the low rate reported to IgG-NMO autoantibody in r-NMO Caribbean patients, it may downregulate cytokine (TNF-α and IL-10) serum levels, causing a worse course of the disease [3, 6]. Here, we explored the influence of IgG-NMO autoantibody on serum S100β levels and clinical events in rNMO Cuban patients.

Material and Methods

Serum samples from 24 patients (age: 38.7 ± 10.13; gender: 23 females/1 male) diagnosed as rNMO according to Winherchuk et al. [7] were tested. Inclusion criteria evidenced no relapse or any immunomodulatory or immunosuppressor treatment, at least 30 days before the test. Ten healthy donors, matched with patients in terms of age and gender, were also evaluated. Written informed consent was collected from each subject. The study followed the Code of Ethical Principles for Medical Research on humans. Clinical and disability data included disease duration (years), annual relapse rate and EDSS (Expanded Disability Status Scale) at last follow-up. This last measure was according to Kurtzke [8].

IgG-NMO Autoantibody Analysis

IgG-NMO autoantibody serum detection was performed by the indirect immunofluorescence assay described by Lennon et al. [9].

ELISA

Evaluation of S100β quantification levels was performed using commercially available luminescence immunoassay (LIAISON Sangtec 100, Byk-Sangtec, Germany) following the manufacturer's instructions.

Statistical Analyses

Data are showed as mean ± SD. Due to the non-gaussian distribution and small sample size, we used Mann-Whitney U tests. Spearman's rank correlation test was used to the correlate the analysis between variables. Statistically significant data were taken at $p < 0.05$.

Results

Clinical and disability data from rNMO patients were as follows: disease duration (8.35 ± 6.4/year), relapse rate/year (0.88 ± 0.73) and EDSS at last follow-up (5.5 ± 2.66). A significant correlation was observed between disability and IgG-NMO ($p = 0.009$). The mean serum concentration of S100β was lower in the rNMO patient group compared to controls, though differences were not significant (table 1). S100β protein levels did not show significant differences regarding IgG-NMO immunoreactivity ($p = 0.82$). S100β levels were similar in patients positive or not to IgG-NMO autoantibody. We did not find any correlation between IgG-NMO and S100β in rNMO.

Discussion

S100β protein binds many intracellular protein targets and modulates cytoskeleton plasticity and cell proliferation [5]. In this study, we found that serum levels of S100β are not correlated to IgG NMO immunoreactivity and disability. These results suggest that serum S100β levels in rNMO patients may not be regulated by IgG-NMO autoantibody. Furthermore, we did not observe any correlation between S100β levels and clinical disability.

One of the limitations of testing S100β plasma levels in neurological disorders in most studies is that there are other sources of this protein besides neurons and glial cells. In fact, it was found that fat tissue, skin and cartilage can release this protein.

Higher levels of the S100β glial marker were found in primary and secondary progressive multiple sclerosis (MS), and also in relapsing-remitting MS during acute stage of the disease [10]. This report could support our results since our patients were not in a relapsing stage at the time of sample collection.

This study also confirms that S100β dysregulation in rNMO is most probably related to an inflammatory activity though it may not be suitable to evidence disability, since it is mainly related to neurodegenerative changes. No correlation to disability was found in this group of patients. At the same time, our findings suggest that rNMO patients might be exhibiting a milder inflammatory process than that seen in other forms of MS. Likewise, they could reflect that serum S100β would be ineffective as a surrogate marker, at least in this state of the disease.

We conclude that IgG-NMO may differentially regulate S100β protein and disability in r-NMO patients and results confirm a diagnostic and probably a prognostic value of the autoantibody to this disease. It would be valuable to identify other surrogate biological markers that are much more dependent on neuropathology such as axonal loss and regeneration.

Acknowledgements

The NMO-IgG autoantibody test was supported by the Fondo de Investigaciones Sanitarias, Madrid, Spain (P1 60070 AS, PG). S100β protein determination was granted by funds of the Biochemical Department, Instituto de Ciências Básicas da Saúde, Universidade Federal do Rio Grande do Sul, Porto Alegre, Brazil. The authors also thank the collaboration of Prof. Cabrera-Gómez, MD, PhD; Lic, Grass Fernandez D. and Lic, Cristófol-Corominas M., Associate Professor.

References

1 Jarius S, Aboul-Enein F, Waters P, et al: Antibody to aquaporin-4 in the long-term course of neuromyelitis optica. Brain 2008; 131:3072–3080.

2 Argyriou AA, Makris N: Neuromyelitis optica: a distinct demyelinating disease of the central nervous system. Acta Neurol Scand 2008;118:209–217.

3 Pentón-Rol G, Cervantes-Llanio M, Martinez-Sasnchez G, Cabrera-Gómez JA, Valenzuela-Silva CM, Ramirez-Nuñez O, Casanova-Orta M, Robinson-Agramonte MA, Lopategui-Cabezas I, Lopez-Saura A: TNF-α and IL-10 downregulation and marked oxidative stress in neuromyelitis optica. J Inflamm 2009;6:18–27.

4 Takano R, Tatsuro M, Toshiyuki T, Masahiro I, Kazuo F, Yasuto I: A prominent elevation of glial fibrillary acidic protein in the cerebrospinal fluid during relapse in neuromyelitis optica. Tohoku J Exp Med 2008;215: 55–59.

5 Van Eldik LJ, Wainwright MS: The Janus face of glial-derived S100B: beneficial and detrimental functions in the brain. Restor Neurol Neurosci 2003;21:97–108.

6 Cabrera-Gomez JA, Bonnan M, González-Quevedo A, Saiz-Hinarejos A, Marignier R, Olindo S, Graus F, Smadja D, Merle H, Thomas L, Gomez-García A, Cabre P: Neuromyelitis optica positive autoantibodies confer a worse course in relapsing-neuromyelitis optica in Cuba and French West India. Mult Scler 2009;15:828–833.

7 Winherchuk DM, Lennon VA, Pittock SJ, Lucchinetti CF, Weinshenker BG: Revised diagnostic criteria for neuromyelitis óptica. Neurology 2006;66:1485–1489.

8 Kurtzke JF: Rating neurologic impairment in multiple sclerosis: an expanded disability status scale (EDSS). Neurology 1083;33: 1444–1452.

9 Jarius S, Aboul-Enein F, Waters P, et al: Antibody to aquaporin-4 in the long-term course of neuromyelitis optica. Brain 2008; 131:3072–3080.

10 Lennon VA, Wingerchuck DM, Kryzer TJ, et al: A serum autoantibody marker of neuromyelitis optica distinction from multiple sclerosis. Lancet 2004;364:2106–2112.

11 Marenholz I, Heizmann CW, Fritz G: S100 proteins in mouse and man: from evolution to function and pathology (including an update of the nomenclature). Biochem Biophys Res Commun 2004;322:1111–1122.

NeuroImmunoModulation

Neuroimmunomodulation 2010;17:180–183
DOI: 10.1159/000258718

Published online: February 4, 2010

Role of Toll-Like Receptors and Inflammation in Adrenal Gland Insufficiency

Waldemar Kanczkowski[a] Kai Zacharowski[b] Stefan R. Bornstein[a]

[a]Department of Medicine III, Carl Gustav Carus University Hospital, Dresden, and [b]Clinic of Anaesthesiology, Intensive Care Medicine and Pain Therapy, Frankfurt, Germany

Key Words
Adrenal damage · Pro-inflammatory cytokines · Adrenal hemorrhage · Pattern recognition receptors · Adrenalitis

Abstract
Adrenal gland insufficiency – the clinical manifestation of deficient production or action of adrenal steroids – is a life-threatening disorder. Among many factors which can predispose to primary adrenal failure, an autoimmune adrenalitis and infectious agents play a major role. The initial host defense against bacterial infections is executed primarily by the pattern recognition receptors, e.g. Toll-like receptors (TLRs), expressed in cells from the innate immune system. Upon activation, TLRs have been found to regulate various levels of innate and adaptive immunity as well as control tissue inflammation. TLRs are implicated in adrenal cell turnover and steroidogenesis during inflammation. Therefore, TLRs play a crucial role in the activation of adrenal inflammation mediating adrenal gland dysfunction during septicemia.

Introduction

Adrenal gland insufficiency – the clinical manifestation or deficient production of action of glucocorticoids, mineralocorticoids and sex hormones – is a life-threatening disorder that requires prompt clinical management. Insufficiency in adrenal gland steroid production may result from either primary adrenal failure including organ damage or secondary adrenal diseases due to impairment of the hypothalamic-pituitary axis [1].

Symptoms of primary adrenal gland insufficiency as first described in 1855 by Thomas Addison are weakness, fatigue, anorexia, and abdominal pain, with orthostatic hypotension, salt craving, and characteristic hyperpigmentation of the skin. Although the prevalence of so-called Addison's disease (AD) in the general population is low, ranging from 60 up to 117 cases per million, the number of newly diagnosed cases increases annually. Because the full manifestation of the AD occurs when 90% of the adrenocortical cells are destroyed, the real number of affected individuals may be underestimated. The main cause of the primary adrenal gland failure, besides of genetic factors, is inflammation [2].

Toll-like receptors (TLRs) are critical components of innate immune system. They play an essential role in host defense by eliciting rapid inflammatory reactions and or-

KARGER

Fax +41 61 306 12 34
E-Mail karger@karger.ch
www.karger.com

1021–7401/10/0173–0180$26.00/0

Accessible online at:
www.karger.com/nim

Waldemar Kanczkowski, Department of Medicine III
Carl Gustav Carus Medical School, University of Technology
Fetscherstrasse 74, DE–01307 Dresden (Germany)
Tel. +49 351 458 6606, Fax +49 351 458 6336
E-Mail waldemar.kanczkowski@uniklinikum-dresden.de

chestrating adaptive innate response to microbial infection. When activated, e.g. during infections, TLRs induce pro-inflammatory cytokine and chemokine synthesis which mediate a rapid recruitment of the leukocytes into the infected tissues. In order to eliminate pathogens, leukocytes release toxic components of their granules including reactive oxygen species (ROS), nitrogen species or, e.g., proteinases. When the acute inflammatory response fails to eliminate the pathogen, or in the case of autoimmune reaction, the inflammatory process persists and results in collateral damage to the host tissues [3].

This article describes the particular role that inflammation plays in adrenal gland insufficiency with a special focus on TLRs.

Adrenal Gland Insufficiency Related to Inflammation

Among many factors known to affect the adrenal gland such as hereditary disorders, drugs and certain diseases, inflammation plays a special role in the pathogenesis of the adrenal gland. In particular, patients with high risk of developing adrenal gland failure are those with multi-organ autoimmune diseases associated with polyendocrinopathy syndrome (APS) type 1 and type 2, persons with tuberculosis or AIDS-associated cytomegalovirus (CMV) infection and finally critically ill patients with septic shock [1].

In developed countries, autoimmune AD is a main cause of primary adrenocortical failure, accounting for nearly 80% of the cases. Clinically, AD often occurs in association with other organ-specific autoimmune disorders such as Hashimoto's thyroid disease, Graves' disease or autoimmune gastritis that are known as APS type 1 and type 2. Although the genetic background and etiology of these syndromes are remarkably different, they both result in a similar autoimmune destruction of the adrenal cortex. The initiation of the pathogenesis of both syndromes is due to a mutation in one of two genes, namely AIRE (autoimmune regulator) for APS1 or CTLA4 (cytotoxic T lymphocyte-associated antigen 4) for APS2. The prevalence of autoreactive antibodies in AD patients is estimated as 50–90%. The latter antibodies react with P450 enzymes involved in steroid synthesis, 21-hydroxylase (P450c21), 17α-hydroxylase (P450c17) and cholesterol side chain-cleaving enzyme (P450scc). Because P450 enzymes are located within mitochondria, the question is whether auto-antibodies are the cause or the consequence of adrenal destruction. Although the mechanism of autoimmune AD is not clear yet, the strong association with an inflammatory process has been documented. Therefore, several components of the immune system, including T cells, autoantibody and complement, are involved in the pathogenesis of adrenocortical destruction. In early stages of the AD disease the adrenal glands may be enlarged with extensive lymphocytic infiltration. When disease progresses, the adrenal gland becomes atrophic and a strong mononuclear infiltration (mainly lymphocytes but also plasma cells and macrophages) is found [2].

In developing countries and in the case of the immunocompromised patients, infections persist as a main cause of the primary adrenal gland dysfunction. Adrenalitis caused either by tuberculosis or CMV infection is often characterized by strong lymphocytic infiltration (mostly $CD8^+$ T cells) as well as upregulation of many proinflammatory cytokines. Studies using modern diagnostic methods such as computer tomography (CT) revealed that during active tuberculosis, patients usually develop bilateral adrenal gland enlargement with or without calcification. Postmortem histological examination of infected adrenal slices reveals usually a tissue necrosis and mixed inflammatory infiltrate [4]. Considering that almost 2 billion people worldwide are infected with *Mycobacterium tuberculosis*, a pathogen causing tuberculosis, the chances that some of them will develop adrenal failure during various forms of immune deficiency are high. Similarly to tuberculosis, CMV-induced adrenalitis is also common in patients with AIDS and is usually characterized by focal necrosis and inflammation of the adrenal gland [5].

Adrenal gland impairment is often found in critically ill patients with systemic inflammatory response syndrome and also as a consequence of septic shock. In these patients adrenal gland failure may either be characterized by inadequate glucocorticoid activity in relation to the severity of the patient's illness or manifests itself as a pathogen-induced adrenal hemorrhage. Since the first syndrome is often related to overt cytokine production and dysregulation of immunoadrenal cross talk, the second is frequently manifested as Waterhouse-Friderichsen syndrome and can be directly induced by pathogens. Symptoms of the Waterhouse-Friderichsen syndrome are sudden onset, short course, fever, cyanosis, patching of the skin and mucous membranes, collapse and coma as a result of bilateral adrenal hemorrhage. Despite being mostly associated with meningococcemia, adrenal hemorrhage may also occur after infection with other pathogens including staphylococci [6].

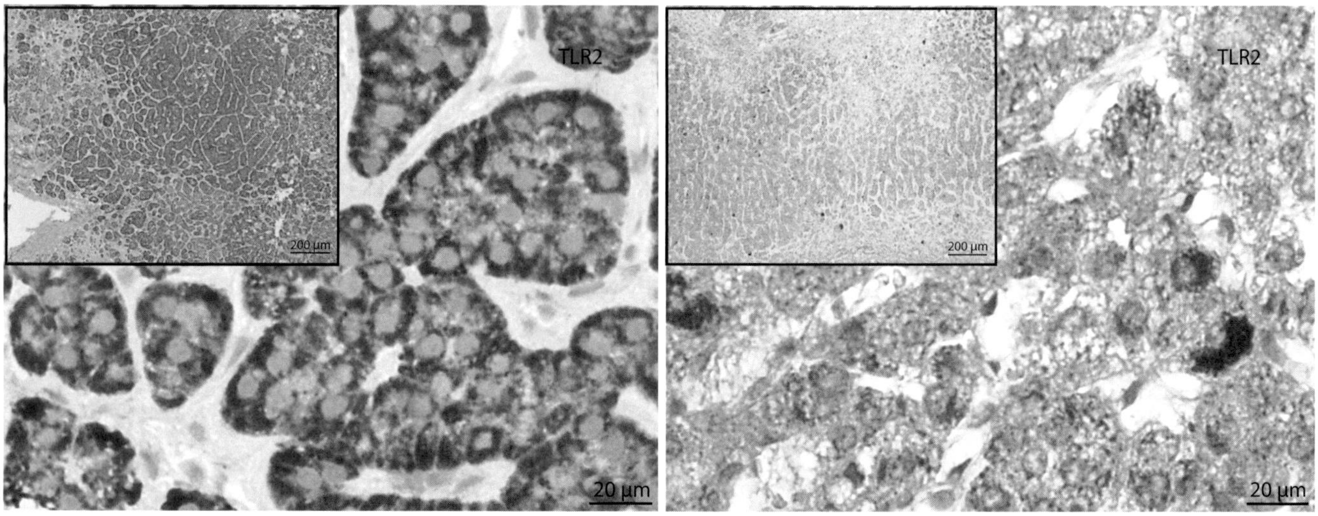

Fig. 1. TLR upregulation in the human adrenal gland during sepsis. Immunohistochemical staining results of human adrenal section showing TLR2 expression of septic adrenal glands (septic patient) and in normal adrenal gland (control patient). The signal was visualized using avidin-biotin labeling and 3,3′-diaminobenzidine. Scale bars are inserted into the right corner and represent 20 μm for main picture and 200 μm for low magnification picture situated at the left upper corner.

Role of TLRs in Adrenal Gland Insufficiency and Damage

TLRs are type I transmembrane pattern recognition receptors which are known to regulate various aspects of innate immunity including an inflammatory reaction related to tissue damage or infections. In order to perform their functions, TLRs are located mainly at the cellular membrane but also in the intracellular compartments where they sense various conserved pathogen-associated molecules. The fine examples of TLRs ligands are Gram-negative bacterial endotoxins such as lipopolysaccharide (LPS) sensed by TLR4, or Gram-positive bacterial lipoproteins, e.g. lipoteichonic acid detected by TLR2. Due to their specific localization, TLRs present in the intracellular compartments recognize microbial patterns such as bacterial or viral DNA (TLR9) or RNA (TLR3 and TLR8). To date, 13 TLRs have been found in mammals and activation of all of them induces strong proinflammatory cytokine responses. Due to their ability to initiate an overt inflammation, TLRs are often associated with destruction of various tissues, e.g. during septic shock. Using TLR-deficient animals or TLR antagonists, a direct correlation between hyperactivation of certain TLR and pathogenesis of several diseases including a stroke, diabetes mellitus, obesity, cardiovascular diseases or autoimmune Hashimoto's disease has been found [3].

TLRs may be involved in the pathogenesis of adrenal gland in many ways. First, during acute or chronic bacterial or viral infections, a strong systemic and local cytokine response is evoked via TLRs expressed in the immune cells, resulting in the alterations of an immunoadrenal cross talk. Furthermore, bacterial and viral infections have been documented to directly impair adrenal gland steroidogenesis, e.g. during adenoviral infection [7]. Moreover, a direct binding of LPS to the surface of adrenocortical cells has been shown by flow-cytometry and was associated with decreased basal and ACTH-induced cortisol production. Further experiments have demonstrated an increased production of ROS which may be the mechanism of the latter observation [8]. Recent data obtained in our laboratory suggest that the negative effect of LPS on adrenocortical cell steroidogenesis could be mediated via TLR4 expressed in steroid-producing cells. Furthermore, we have demonstrated that adrenocortical cells also express other members of the TLR family, which sensitize these cells to pathogenic action [9]. Moreover, we found that TLR2, TLR4 or TLR9 ligands when administered to mice induce a strong systemic and local inflammation of adrenal gland with upregulation of the major proinflammatory cytokines such as IL-1, IL-6 and TNF-α [10]. Besides the strong induction of cytokines [9], TLR ligands have been found to directly cause adrenocortical cell apoptosis as well as promote adrenal gland hemorrhage in animal models [11]. The induction of adrenal inflammation is often paralleled with an upregulation of TLR expression, both in vivo and in vitro. A strong upregulation of TLR2 expression can be shown in the adrenal glands of septic patients that directly links adrenal gland damage with TLR overexpression (fig. 1). Although not yet demonstrated in adrenal gland, overstimulation of TLR3 in thyroid gland results in the inflammation and initiation of an autoimmune thyroiditis [12]. Surprisingly, unlike in other organs in which deficiency of one of the TLRs was shown to prevent or limit organ damage during inflammation, e.g. in the brain, TLR2 and TLR4 deficiency in adrenal gland results in an impaired adrenal glucocorticoid stress response. Moreover, TLR deficiency results in an impairment of the ultrastructure of the adrenocortical cells indicating a novel role of TLR in the adrenal gland apart from the regulation of the immunoadrenal cross talk [10].

Summarizing, inflammation resulted either from an autoimmune process or, being a part of antimicrobial defense, is associated with adrenal gland insufficiency. The hyperactivation of TLRs in both immune and adrenocortical cells is involved in the pathogenesis of the adrenal gland. Therefore, a development of new treatments and drugs which can antagonize TLR signaling is expected in the future. Results obtained from TLR-deficient mice, however, clearly suggest that a careful monitoring of adrenal gland function during such therapy is necessary.

Acknowledgment

This work was supported by a grant from the 'Deutsche Forschungsgemeinschaft' to S.R.B. (BO 1141-8-2).

References

1 Bornstein SR: Predisposing factors for adrenal insufficiency. N Engl J Med 2009;360: 2328–2339.
2 Martin MP, Roep BO, Smit JW: Autoimmunity in Addison's disease. Neth J Med 2002; 60:269–275.
3 Gay NJ, Gangloff M: Structure and function of Toll receptors and their ligands. Annu Rev Biochem 2007;76:141–165.
4 Wang L, Yang J: Tuberculous Addison's disease mimics malignancy in FDG-PET images. Intern Med 2008;47:1755–1756.
5 Price P, Olver SD, Silich M, et al: Adrenalitis and the adrenocortical response of resistant and susceptible mice to acute murine cytomegalovirus infection. Eur J Clin Invest 1996;26:811–819.
6 Hamilton D, Harris MD, Foweraker J, et al: Waterhouse-Friderichsen syndrome as a result of non-meningococcal infection. J Clin Pathol 2004;57:208–209.
7 Alesci S, Ramsey WJ, Bornstein SR, et al: Adenoviral vectors can impair adrenocortical steroidogenesis: clinical implications for natural infections and gene therapy. Proc Natl Acad Sci USA 2002;99:7484–7489.
8 Garcia R, Enriquez de SA, Portoles MT: Calcium and reactive oxygen species as messengers in endotoxin action on adrenocortical cells. Biochim Biophys Acta 1999;1454–1464.
9 Kanczkowski W, Zacharowski K, Wirth MP, et al: Differential expression and action of Toll-like receptors in human adrenocortical cells. Mol Cell Endocrinol 2009;300:57–65.
10 Zacharowski K, Zacharowski PA, Koch A, et al: Toll-like receptor 4 plays a crucial role in the immune-adrenal response to systemic inflammatory response syndrome. Proc Natl Acad Sci USA 2006;103:6392–6397.
11 Levin J, Cluff LE: Endotoxemia and adrenal hemorrhage: a mechanism for the Waterhouse-Friderichsen syndrome. J Exp Med 1965;121:247–260.
12 Harii N, Lewis CJ, Vasko V, et al: Thyrocytes express a functional toll-like receptor 3: overexpression can be induced by viral infection and reversed by phenylmethimazole and is associated with Hashimoto's autoimmune thyroiditis. Mol Endocrinol 2005;19: 1231–1250.

NeuroImmunoModulation

Neuroimmunomodulation 2010;17:184–187
DOI: 10.1159/000258719

Published online: February 4, 2010

A Clinical Correlate of the Dysregulated Immunoendocrine Response in Human Tuberculosis

Natalia Santucci[a] Luciano D'Attilio[a] Hugo Besedovsky[b] Adriana del Rey[b] María Luisa Bay[a] Oscar Bottasso[a]

[a]Instituto de Inmunología, Facultad de Ciencias Médicas, Universidad Nacional de Rosario, Rosario, Argentina;
[b]Institute of Physiology and Pathophysiology, Marburg, Germany

Key Words

Tuberculosis · Adrenal steroids · Cytokines · Leptin

Abstract

Wasting is a prominent feature in tuberculosis (TB), but its underlying mechanisms are incompletely understood. Immunoendocrine disturbances may be linked to the consumption state of TB patients, since hormones and cytokines can affect energy expenditure and metabolism. To approach this possibility, we have determined leptin, IL-18, and adrenal steroid plasma levels and body mass index (BMI) in newly diagnosed patients with mild, moderate and severe pulmonary TB, household contacts (HHC), and healthy controls (HCO). HHC displayed higher levels of leptin than HCO and TB patients. TB patients showed a gradual decrease in BMI and leptin concentrations with increasing disease severity, whereas a positive correlation between this hormone and BMI was found in the HCO group. Cortisol concentrations tended to be higher in TB patients. DHEA levels were decreased in TB patients and to a lesser extent in HHC, whereas IL-18 concentration was significantly increased in patients with severe disease. Since HHC are known to cause a latent subclinical infection, it seems clear that controlled tuberculous infection and manifested TB disease are accompanied by a dissimilar profile of immunoendocrine markers.

Host defense against microbial pathogens is carried out by innate and acquired immune mechanisms. The initial detection and the immune response to microbial infection relies to great extent on a family of pattern recognition receptors, resulting in a chain of signaling events necessary to kill the pathogens, in addition to promoting the initiation of adaptive immune responses.

The inflammation usually accompanying these processes is a temporary and self-limiting response essential to restore tissue homeostasis and the subsequent healing processes. When the pathogen cannot be controlled by the initial immunoinflammatory response, a systemic response follows. This response induces multiple metabolic and neuroendocrine changes [1], leading to profound alterations in homeostasis that support host defense. There is growing evidence that chronic inflammation is the expression of immune dysregulation, characterized by a state of sustained immune reactivity in the presence of persistence and/or progression of a disease process. In this way, increasing tissue damage followed by unsuccessful tissue repair may result in breaking self-tolerance, malignant transformation, fibrotic changes and metabolic alterations [2].

Immune cells are functionally active within adipose tissue exerting potent effects on adipocyte metabolism and endocrine function. In turn, the adipose tissue constitutes an active secretory organ, sending and respond-

KARGER

Fax +41 61 306 12 34
E-Mail karger@karger.ch
www.karger.com

1021–7401/10/0173–0184$26.00/0

Accessible online at:
www.karger.com/nim

Dr. Oscar Bottasso
Instituto de Inmunología, Facultad de Ciencias Médicas
Universidad Nacional de Rosario, Santa Fe 3100
Rosario 2000 (Argentina)
Tel. +54 341 480 4559, Fax +54 341 480 4569, E-Mail bottasso@uolsinectis.com.ar

ing to signals that modulate appetite, energy expenditure, insulin sensitivity, endocrine functions, inflammation and immunity [2]. The contribution of adipose tissue-derived cells to the immune response may play a significant role in host defense mechanisms, underscoring their involvement in an immune response during physiological or pathological conditions. Reasons for a strong relationship between the immune system and energy stores are not fully understood. It is clear that the host needs a reasonably stable energy supply to preserve all biological functions, without affecting some often competing physiological processes. Studies employing a variety of antigenic stimuli in different vertebrate and invertebrate species provided evidence for the energetic costs of immune reactivity [2]. The increased energy dedicated to mount an immune response, adaptive in principle to clear pathogens, can ultimately result in decreased fitness if immune activation becomes prolonged or excessive due to an inability to control the infection.

Tuberculosis (TB) is a representative example of an abnormal immunoendocrine metabolic relation due to an infection. It constitutes a major health problem worldwide and can lead to a consumption state, characterized by a remarkable weight loss [3, 4], traditionally defined as cachexia (Greek *kakos* = bad and *hexis* = condition). Because of its chronic nature, the disease is accompanied by excessive and/or protracted cytokine production liable to affect the immunoendocrine communication [3]. Our studies in TB patients showed increased IFN-γ, IL-10, and IL-6 plasma levels in the presence of modest increases in cortisol, prolactin and thyroid hormones and highly augmented concentrations of growth hormone. In contrast, testosterone and dehydroepiandrosterone (DHEA) levels were decreased [3]. There is reason to believe that the consumption state of TB patients is linked to the immunoendocrine disturbances, given the role of immune and endocrine mediators in energy expenditure and metabolism. We have demonstrated that the body mass index (BMI) is negatively associated with circulating IL-6 levels in patients with active TB. Stepwise regression analysis showed that 74% of the variability in IL-6 concentration was related to BMI, cortisol and IFN-γ serum concentrations [4]. Adjusted analysis also showed that impaired in vitro immune responses of these TB patients (reduced lymphoproliferation and increased IL-10 and TGF-β production) lost statistically significance when adjusted to their BMI. These results reinforce the view of the intricate relation between the immunoendocrine imbalance and consumption state, further affecting the anti-infective immune response.

Several mechanisms acting simultaneously may account for these findings. An association between increased IL-6 concentrations and loss of appetite was found in TB patients [5]. Furthermore, decreased levels of testosterone, a powerful anabolic hormone, are expected to contribute to a reduction of the BMI.

Nevertheless, it is now clear that the communication between the metabolic state and the immune response also involves products released by the adipose tissue that modulate appetite, energy expenditure, insulin sensitivity, endocrine and reproductive systems, inflammation and immunity. Hence, wasting during TB may be the result of a more complex and imbalanced relation among pro-inflammatory cytokines, hormones and neuropeptides involved in feeding control and adipocytokines, like leptin.

Determinations of plasma leptin in TB patients yielded dissimilar results. While some reports showed increased leptin levels in TB patients [6], they were found decreased in another study in which they were also associated with body fat and loss of appetite [7]. Schwenk et al. [8] suggest that leptin is not involved in the loss of weight and appetite in TB, although in their study leptin correlated with body mass. Since a tissue granulomatous reaction is observed in tuberculosis together with weight loss, and leptin is involved in both metabolism and the immune response, it is difficult to discern to what extent leptin levels are related to an energy imbalance or to the chronic immune process underlying the infection. Studies on the immunoendocrine metabolic relation in household contacts (HHC) of TB patients may be informative since these individuals undergo a latent subclinical tuberculous infection (LTBI), show no consumption, and share the same socioeconomic and environmental conditions. A study in 48 newly diagnosed patients with pulmonary TB (11 mild, 19 moderate, 18 severe), 20 HHC, and 29 healthy controls (HCO) was carried out to analyze plasma leptin, adrenal steroids, and IL-18 levels and BMI. All subjects were HIV negative and were comparable in age and sex distribution (58 females, 39 males, overall mean $\pm$ SEM age 39 $\pm$ 1.9 years). HHC displayed higher levels of leptin than controls and TB patients (table 1). Furthermore, TB patients showed a gradual decrease in leptin concentrations with increasing disease severity, whereas a positive correlation between this hormone and BMI was found in the HCO group ($p < 0.05$). Cortisol concentrations tended to be higher in TB patients. Levels of DHEA were decreased in TB patients and to a lesser extent in HHC, respect the HCO group ($p < 0.01$). IL-18 concentration was significantly increased in patients with severe disease ($p < 0.05$).

Table 1. Plasma concentrations of leptin, cortisol, DHEA and IL-18 and BMI in the study groups

Groups	Leptin, ng/ml	Cortisol, ng/ml	DHEA, ng/ml	IL-18, pg/ml	BMI
Controls (n = 28)	11.6 ± 1.92	115 ± 11.4	11 ± 2.53**	247.4 ± 41.4	27 ± 1.19***
HHC (n = 20)	16.9 ± 3.17#	106 ± 51.8	5.84 ± 4.4	231 ± 31.7	27.9 ± 6.6***
Mild (n = 11)	6.81 ± 2.54	97.4 ± 14.5	4.27 ± 2	345 ± 104	22.3 ± 0.76
Moderate (n = 18)	3.98 ± 1.33*	130 ± 13.1	4.16 ± 0.75	367 ± 109.8	22.9 ± 1.16
Severe (n = 18)	3.58 ± 1.56*	122 ± 62	3.89 ± 1	517 ± 69.9‡	20.8 ± 1.58

Data represent means ± SEM and are statistically analyzed by the Kruskal-Wallis and Mann-Whitney U tests. * Significantly different from controls, $p < 0.05$. # Significantly different from mild, moderate and severe patients, $p < 0.05$. ** Significantly different from the remaining groups, $p < 0.01$. *** Significantly different from the three groups of TB patients, $p < 0.01$. ‡ Significantly different from HHC and HCO, $p < 0.05$.

Taken together with our studies showing that HHC mount a strong cell-mediated immune response to mycobacteria indicating a LTBI [9], it can be assumed that controlled or progressive tuberculous infection coexist with two different types of immuno-endocrine relations. In fact, tuberculosis is accompanied by weight loss, decreased leptin and DHEA levels, and increased IL-18 concentrations, whereas no weight loss, normal to augmented leptin, unchanged IL-18 and decreased DHEA levels are seen in HHC.

Leptin constitutes a crucial link between immunity and nutrition as it reduces food intake, augments energy expenditure, favor Th1 responses, and production of several pro-inflammatory cytokines by monocytes/macrophages [10]. Reduced leptin levels in TB patients may be partly due to the wasting accompanying the disease. The fact that reduced leptin levels coexist with the typical anorexia these patients present seems paradoxical. Nevertheless, it should be noted that inflammatory mediators released during acute infections increase leptin synthesis, whereas chronic stimulation with proinflammatory cytokines, as is the case of TB, suppresses its production [10]. Confirming earlier observations [3], DHEA was also decreased in TB patients. Since DHEA stimulates T helper cell functions, facilitates Th1 responses and also displays potent anti-inflammatory effects [3], its reduction seems to be harmful for the course of the disease. Regarding IL-18, this cytokine exerts pleiotropic effects both during innate and adaptive immune responses [11]. It possesses powerful inflammatory properties and widespread immune-augmenting functions. For example, in the presence of IL-12, IL-18 drives the Th1 polarization and is protective during experimental TB [12], whereas in the absence of IL-12, IL-18 promotes Th2 differentiation [11]. Considering the effects of IL-18 on Th1 responses, increased levels of this cytokine in TB patients, which are more evident in those with progressive disease, suggest that IL-18 is devoid of Th1-promoting effects during TB, probably being mostly pro-inflammatory.

Close contacts of active TB patients are most likely to course a LTBI. Contrasting increased levels of leptin in HHC in the presence of a preserved and somehow augmented BMI may be due to a subpatent inflammation accompanying a LTBI. Reduced DHEA levels in HHC may be also related to immune mechanisms triggered by LTBI, since we have previously shown that supernatants from cultures of antigen-specific stimulated mononuclear cells from TB patients inhibit DHEA production by adrenal cells [3]. Nevertheless, HHC can mount a strong cell-mediated immune response when stimulated with mycobacterial antigens [9], suggesting the presence of a compensatory mechanism despite the diminished levels of DHEA.

Cross-sectional studies are limited in terms of causation, since potential predictors and end points are measured at the same time. Nevertheless, these preliminary results add new information to the profile of immuno-endocrine alterations present in TB patients, being clear that leptin concentrations may distinguish a reasonably immunoprotective status from an immunopathological condition. Attempts are now being made to expand the analysis of mediators involved in the immuno-endocrine-metabolic unit to get a more integrative view of the complex mechanisms underlying TB pathophysiology.

Acknowledgements

The present study received financial support from FONCYT (research grant BID 1728/OC-AR 5-25462) and Fundación Florencio Fiorini.

References

1 Besedovsky H, del Rey A: Immune-neuro-endocrine interactions: facts and hypothesis. Endocr Rev 1996;17:64–95.
2 Bottasso O, Docena G, Stanford JL, Grange JM: Chronic inflammation as a manifestation of defects in immunoregulatory networks: implications for novel therapies based on microbial products. Inflammopharmacology 2009;17:193–203.
3 del Rey A, Mahuad CV, Bozza V, Bogue C, Farroni MA, Bay ML, Bottasso OA, Besedovsky HO: Endocrine and cytokine responses in humans with pulmonary tuberculosis. Brain Behav Immun 2007;21:171–179.
4 Mahuad C, Bozza V, Pezzotto SM, Bay ML, Besedovsky H, del Rey A, Bottasso O: Impaired immune responses in tuberculosis patients are related to weight loss that coexists with an immunoendocrine imbalance. Neuroimmunomodulation 2007;14:193–199.
5 van Lettow M, van der Meer JWM, West CE, van Crevel R, Semba RD: Interleukin-6 and human immunodeficiency virus load, nut not plasma leptin concentration, predict anorexia and wasting in adults with pulmonary tuberculosis in Malawi. J Clin Endocrinol Metab 2005;90:4771–4776.
6 Yuksel I, Sencan M, Dokmetas HS, Dokmetas I, Ataseven H, Yonem A: The relation between serum leptin levels and body fat mass in patients with active lung tuberculosis. Endocr Res 2003;29:257–264.
7 van Crevel R, Karyadi E, Netea MG, Verhoef H, Nelwan RH, West CE, van der Meer JW: Decreased plasma leptin concentrations in tuberculosis patients are associated with wasting and inflammation. J Clin Endocrinol Metab 2002;87:758–763.
8 Schwenk A, Hodgson L, Rayner CFJ, Griffin GE, Macallan DC: Leptin and energy metabolism in pulmonary tuberculosis. Am J Clin Nutr 2003;77:392–398.
9 Bozza V, D'Attilio L, Didoli G, Santucci N, Nannini L, Bogue C, Del Rey A, Besedovsky H, Bay Ml, Bottasso O: The adrenal steroid response during tuberculosis and its effects on the mycobacterial-driven IFN-γ production of patients and their household contacts. Ann NY Acad Sci 2009;1153:247–255.
10 La Cava A, Matarese G: The weight of leptin in immunity. Nat Rev Immunol 2004;4:371–379.
11 Gracie JA, Robertson SE, McInnes IB: Interleukin-18. J Leukoc Biol 2003;73:213–224.
12 Schneider B, Korbel D, Hagens K, Koch M, Raupach B, Enders J, Kaufmann SHE, Mittrucker HW: Interleukin 18 is essential for protective immunity against *Mycobacterium tuberculosis*; in: Tuberculosis, Biology, Pathology and Therapy. Colorado, Keystone Symposia Global Health Series, 2009, p 138, abstr 411.

NeuroImmunoModulation

Neuroimmunomodulation 2010;17:188–191
DOI: 10.1159/000258720

Published online: February 4, 2010

Immune Neuroendocrine Interactions during a Fungal Infection in Immunocompetent or Immunosuppressed Hosts

María Cecilia Rodríguez-Galán Claudia E. Sotomayor Roxana Cano Carina Porporatto María Sol Renna María Gabriela Paraje Hugo Cejas Silvia G. Correa

Immunology, Department of Clinical Biochemistry, CIBICI (CONICET), Faculty of Chemical Sciences, National University of Cordoba, Cordoba, Argentina

Key Words
Fungal infection · Stress · Liver · Steatosis

Abstract
The yeast *Candida albicans* belongs to the microflora of healthy individuals, although it can infect a variety of tissues ensuing changes in the host's immune status. To evaluate the effect of neuroendocrine input on the early immune response during the fungal infection, we use a 3-day paradigm of chronic varied stress in Wistar rats infected with *C. albicans*. We find that stress mediators contribute to the spread of the fungus and downregulate critical functions of phagocytic cells at the infection site. Phenotypic and functional alterations of effector cells account for the decreased resistance to candidiasis and condition the development of the adaptive response. Stressed hosts exhibit a higher fungal burden in kidneys and livers associated with hyphal forms. The hepatic inflammatory reaction is compromised with severe steatosis, increment of functional enzymes, marked lipid peroxidation and hepatocyte apoptosis. Moreover, infection-related sickness symptoms are significantly increased by exposure to stress with anorexia, weight loss, lack of leptin and depletion of glycogen depots. Food deprivation exacerbates the liver injury. Stress mediators perturb the complex immune and metabolic program that operates early during fungal spread and promotes severe tissue damage.

Candida albicans is both a constituent of the normal microbiota and a pathogen of humans that can infect a wide range of body sites. This prototypic opportunistic yeast is able to persistently colonize the host without causing symptoms. The balance between commensalism and pathogenicity is an active process and the impairment of the host immunocompetence is considered one major predisposing factor [1]. *C. albicans* infections increased dramatically in the last decades associated to the use of broad spectrum antibiotics, endocrine disorders, tumors or AIDS highlighting the connection between candidiasis and immunocompetence. To evaluate the effect of the neuroendocrine input on the early immune response during the fungal infection, we developed a model of infection and stress in Wistar rats. For the infection, we injected i.p. 3×10^8 viable *C. albicans* cells and we started the stress exposure immediately after infection (IS group) [2]. The stress paradigm lasted 3 days and

KARGER

Fax +41 61 306 12 34
E-Mail karger@karger.ch
www.karger.com

1021–7401/10/0173–0188$26.00/0

Accessible online at:
www.karger.com/nim

Silvia G. Correa
Immunology, Department of Clinical Biochemistry, CIBICI (CONICET)
Faculty of Chemical Sciences, National University of Cordoba
Haya de la Torre y Medina Allende, Cordoba 5000 (Argentina)
Tel. +54 351 434 4973, Fax +54 351 433 3048, E-Mail scorrea@bioclin.fcq.unc.edu.ar

included cold swimming, restraint and food deprivation [2, 3]. Additionally, uninfected unstressed (N), stressed (S) or infected (I) groups were included as controls. Rats were weighed daily and killed after 3 days of treatment to obtain blood and tissues for different studies. We found a significant increment in the levels of ACTH and corticosterone in the IS group, in agreement with the sustained input of the hypothalamus-pituitary-adrenal axis [2, 4]. We observed increments in liver and spleen weights in both infected (I and IS) groups, although the thymus size remained unchanged. A similar fungal burden was detected in the kidneys and spleens of infected rats, whereas livers were heavily colonized in infected stressed hosts. Stained liver sections showed budding yeasts enclosed inside large and well-developed granulomas in I rats [2], whereas invasive hyphae or pseudohyphae forms predominated in IS hosts exhibiting incomplete granulomatous lesions [2, 5]. As TNF-α is crucial for developing a protective inflammatory reaction and antigens of the fungal cell wall induce TNF-α production [6], we evaluated the production of this cytokine under the different experimental conditions. As expected, we detected the highest serum levels of TNF-α in infected hosts on the first day of the infection. Yet, compared with I rats, the IS group showed a 30% lower concentration of the cytokine [7]. On the other hand, on day 3 we found increments in IL-6 and IL-10 levels in I and S groups, respectively. The analysis of liver sections from infected groups showed fat deposition or steatosis [2, 5]. Interestingly, when compared with I rats, livers of IS rats showed a remarkable higher number of fat vacuoles. Hepatic steatosis is caused by imbalance between the delivery of fat in the liver and its subsequent secretion or metabolism; it is a common feature of many liver diseases with different pathogenic mechanisms. To study the distribution and characteristics of steatosis, we stained sections with the specific lipid dye Sudan Black. Strikingly, in I rats microvesicular steatosis predominated all over hepatic acini while in IS group, we detected mainly lipid accumulation in acinar zone 1, with a mixed pattern of micro- and macrosteatosis. While markers of liver injury such as gamma-glutamyl transpeptidase augmented in all treated groups, the intracellular alanine transferase enzyme increased twice in I and IS rats [4]. As steatosis is frequently associated with oxidative stress, we measured the production of malonaldehyde, an indicator of lipid peroxidation. Interestingly, although this marker increased in all treated groups, the highest levels appeared in IS rats. We also evaluated the presence of apoptotic cells on liver sections after staining with the fluorescent dye DAPI. The microscopic analysis showed clear differences in the frequency and nucleus morphology of hepatocytes from the I and IS groups compared with uninfected controls (N and S), with the strongest alterations on day 3 of the treatment [8]. This phenomenon was quantified by TUNEL assay, where apoptotic cells incorporate specifically FITC-labeled dUTP into DNA strand breaks. Again, a significant number of TUNEL-positive cells was found in IS rats compared with I animals ($p < 0.05$). In an attempt to assess the contribution of fungal factors in the liver injury detected in our experimental condition, we identified a 70-kDa lipase that is released after 24 h incubation in standard culture media. This *C. albicans* lipase exhibited maximal activity at physiological pH and temperature and was able to interact with hepatocytes, to induce cytotoxicity and to promote the deposition of lipid droplets [9], replicating the effect observed in vivo. At the peritoneal cavity, the recruitment of leukocytes that occurred after the fungal injection was severely impaired by stress exposure [7]. Whereas the phagocytosis of peritoneal macrophages was not modified, stress mediators decreased the candidicidal activity, evaluated by flow cytometry and killing assay ($p < 0.001$), as well as the production of nitric oxide (NO) [2, 4]. In consequence, the amount of viable *C. albicans* recovered from the peritoneum was significantly higher in IS rats ($p < 0.05$). Together, this first set of studies enabled us to characterize the early innate response during the *C. albicans* infection in immunosuppressed hosts and to conclude that: (1) at the systemic level these rats exhibited a reduction of TNF-α and IL-6 production, poorly developed granulomas, different type and localization of steatosis and severe liver injury, and (2) at the infection site, they showed lower cell recruitment, reduced candidicidal index and higher fungal load.

During an immune response the host needs to organize and distribute energy resources. For that reason, infection is associated with negative energy balance with reduced food intake, weight loss, increased thermogenesis and fever [10]. Then, we wondered how, in our model, hosts exposed to different experimental conditions could achieve the immunometabolic adjustment. Both infection and stress mediators provoked body weight reductions and anorexia, although with different kinetics. By blocking the active TNF-α (with a specific antibody) or corticosterone (with the receptor antagonist RU 486), we reverted the weight loss observed in the IS and I groups, respectively. Leptin is a central mediator that connects nutrition and immunity and regulates satiety. Compared with controls, leptinemia was significantly reduced in all

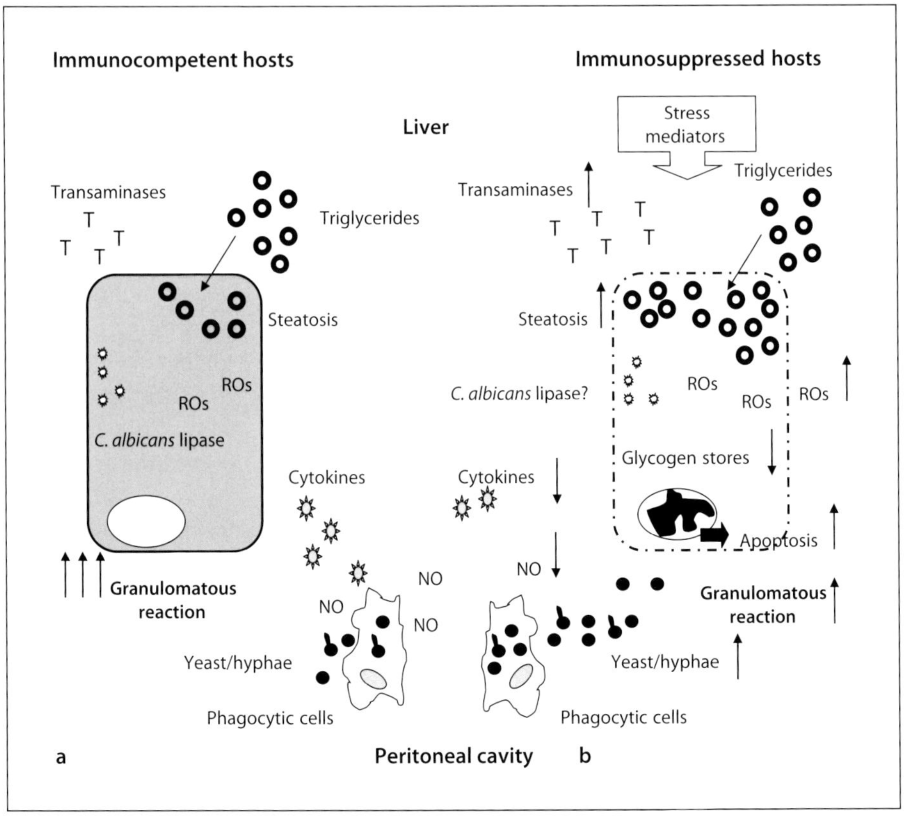

Fig. 1. Outcome of the *C. albicans* infection in immunocompetent or immunosuppressed hosts. Schematic representation of the main biochemical and immune events involved in the early steps of the fungal spreading. The predominant effect of stress mediators on the different parameters evaluated is represented by arrows: ↑ = increment; ↓ = reduction. **a** At the site of the infection, in immunocompetent hosts, the infection activates phagocytic cells that release cytokines such as TNF-α and IL-6 or inflammatory mediators such as NO. The candidicidal mechanisms effectively clear the pathogen significantly reducing spread. In the liver, well-developed granulomas that enclose invasive forms evidence the robust inflammatory reaction. Fungal virulence factors such as *C. albicans* lipase contribute to the fat deposition. Injury markers such as transaminases, lipid peroxidation and microvesicular steatosis are present during the infection although at moderate levels. **b** In the immunosuppressed host, stress mediators severely condition the function of phagocytic cells at the site of the infection. The reduced production of cytokines and NO supports the heavy fungal burden and the higher spreading of invasive hyphal forms. In the liver, the weak inflammatory reaction is evidenced by poorly developed granulomas. Stress mediators could modulate the release of *C. albicans* lipase. Together, in this microenvironment a more severe damage takes place.

treated groups (vs. N, $p < 0.05$) with the stronger reduction in stressed rats. Glycogen stores evaluated in periodic acid-Schiff (PAS)-stained liver sections showed a severe depletion in IS together with a significant reduction in glucose levels ($p < 0.05$). To establish the contribution of food deprivation to the imbalance observed in IS rats, we included two additional experimental groups: (1) rats injected i.p. with 3×10^8 viable *C. albicans* cells as above and exposed to food deprivation on day 2 (IFD group), and (2) rats infected and stressed like the IS group but exposed on day 3 to a 24-hour crowding session instead of food deprivation (ISL group). Clearly, the food deprivation event (IS and IFD) precipitated the complete depletion of glycogen stores and the reduction of glycemia. Steatosis was present in each infected group; however, the highest severity was associated to the stress exposure (IS and ISL). Interestingly, in immunocompetent hosts (IFD), the food deprivation exacerbated the liver injury, with significant increments in lipid peroxidation and transaminase release ($p < 0.05$). We also evaluated the relationship between the ability to clear the fungus and the metabolic imbalance. Compared with immunocompetent hosts, both stressed groups (IS and ISL) showed a higher fungal burden in liver (vs. I, $p < 0.05$) while the single event of food deprivation on day 2 (IFD) was unable to condition the ability of the host to remove the yeast (vs. I, p = n.s.). On the basis of the extensive data presented here, a model of the mechanism involved in the host-fungus interaction in immunocompetent and immunosuppressed hosts can be proposed (fig. 1). In immunocompetent hosts at the site of the infection (i.e. the peritoneal cavity), resident and recruited phagocytic cells become activated and release inflammatory mediators such as NO and cytokines. Different candidicidal mechanisms effectively clear the pathogen significantly reducing the fungal spread (fig. 1a). In the liver, the robust inflammatory reaction is evidenced by well-developed granulomas surrounding invasive forms. The oxidative environment triggers a mild injury in the organ with lipid peroxidation, microvesicular steatosis and transaminase release. Fungal virulence factors such as *C. albicans* lipase could contribute to the fat deposition. In immunosuppressed hosts instead, stress mediators severely condition the function of phagocytic cells at the site of the infection. The impaired release of cytokines and NO promotes the heavier fungal burden and the higher spreading of invasive hyphal forms. In the liver, the weak inflammatory reaction is evidenced by poorly developed granulomas (fig. 1b). Although we have no evidence yet, the modulatory effect of the stress input on the production of *C. albicans* lipase cannot be discarded. Together, the outcome of a fungal infection as well as the liver damage strongly depend on the metabolic and immune status of the host. As defenses are energetically expensive to develop and to operate, the synchronization of inflammatory and metabolic pathways sustains the redistribution of resources under different conditions. Understanding this complex response may help to explain the progression of systemic infections occurring under different metabolic conditions in immunocompromised hosts.

References

1 Hube B: From commensal to pathogen: stage- and tissue-specific gene expression of *Candida albicans*. Curr Opin Microbiol 2004;7:336–341.

2 Rodriguez-Galán MC, Correa SG, Cejas H, Sotomayor CE: Impaired activity of phagocytic cells in *Candida albicans* infection after exposure to chronic varied stress. Neuroimmunomodulation 2001;9:193–202.

3 Correa SG, Rodriguez-Galán MC, Rivero VE, Riera CM: Chronic varied stress modulates experimental autoimmune encephalomyelitis in Wistar rats. Brain Behav Immun 1998;12:134–148.

4 Rodriguez-Galán MC, Sotomayor C, Costamagna ME, Cabanillas AM, Rentería BS, Masini-Repiso AM, Correa S: Immunocompetence of macrophages in rats exposed to *Candida albicans* infection and stress. Am J Physiol Cell Physiol 2003;284:C111–C118.

5 Correa SG, Rodríguez-Galán MC, Salido-Rentería B, Cano R, Cejas H, Sotomayor CE: High dissemination and hepatotoxicity in rats infected with *Candida albicans* after stress exposure: potential sensitization to liver damage. Int Immunol 2004;16:1761–1768.

6 Vazquez N, Buckley HR, Rogers TJ: Production of IL-6 and TNF-alpha by the macrophage-like cell line RAW 264.7 after treatment with a cell wall extract of *Candida albicans*. J Interferon Cytokine Res 1996;16: 465–470.

7 Rodriguez-Galán MC, Correa SG, Iribarren P, Sotomayor CE: Phenotypic and functional changes on phagocytic cells recruited at the site of *Candida albicans* infection after chronic varied stress exposure. Med Mycol 2002;40:485–492.

8 Renna MS, Correa SG, Porporatto C, Figueredo CM, Aoki MP, Paraje MG, Sotomayor CE: Hepatocellular apoptosis during *Candida albicans* colonization: involvement of TNF-alpha and infiltrating Fas-L positive lymphocytes. Int Immunol 2006;18:1719–1728.

9 Paraje MG, Correa SG, Renna MS, Theumer M, Sotomayor CE: *Candida albicans*-secreted lipase induces injury and steatosis in immune and parenchymal cells. Can J Microbiol 2008;54:647–659.

10 Hotamisligil GS, Erbay E: Nutrient sensing and inflammation in metabolic diseases. Nat Rev Immunol 2008;8:923–934.

NeuroImmunoModulation

Neuroimmunomodulation 2010;17:192–195
DOI: 10.1159/000258721

Published online: February 4, 2010

Interplay between Neuroimmunoendocrine Systems during Post-Traumatic Stress Disorder: A Minireview

Moisés E. Bauer[b, c] Andréa Wieck[c] Rodrigo P. Lopes[c, e] Antonio L. Teixeira[d] Rodrigo Grassi-Oliveira[a]

[a]Faculty of Psychology, [b]Faculty of Biosciences, and [c]Institute of Biomedical Research, Pontifical Catholic University of Rio Grande do Sul (PUCRS), Porto Alegre, [d]Department of Internal Medicine, School of Medicine, Federal University of Minas Gerais (UFMG), Belo Horizonte, and [e]BD Biosciences, R. Alexandre Dumas, 1976 – Chácara Santo Antônio, São Paulo, Brazil

Key Words

Post-traumatic stress disorder · Cortisol · Hypocortisolism · Cytokines · Inflammation · Lymphocytes

Abstract

Early life stress has been suggested to mediate vulnerability to affective disorders. Traumatic events experienced in childhood such as sexual abuse and/or physical neglect may lead to psychiatric diseases in adult life, including post-traumatic stress disorder (PTSD). Previous studies have focused on adult traumatic events and very little is known regarding the long-term physiological effects of early life stress. Here, we review the complex interplay between most important cognitive, neuroendocrine and immunological changes reported in PTSD, focusing on long-term implications of childhood maltreatment. PTSD has been associated with significant biological changes related to impaired cognitive functions, attenuated hypothalamic-pituitary-adrenal (HPA) axis function (hypocortisolism) and activation of innate immune responses (low-grade inflammation).

Introduction

Early life stress has been suggested to mediate vulnerability to psychopathology such as major depression and post-traumatic stress disorder (PTSD). Previous studies have mainly focused on adult traumatic events and very little is known regarding the long-term physiological effects of early life stress. Here, we review the complex interplay between cognitive, neuroendocrine and immunological changes reported in PTSD, focusing on long-term implications of childhood maltreatment. We discuss that many biological changes observed during PTSD could be attributable to insufficiency of glucocorticoid signaling.

Impaired HPA Axis Function

There is a general consensus that PTSD is associated with hypocortisolism. This finding may constitute a paradox because ever since the seminal studies by Selye (1936), stress has been associated with activation of the HPA axis with increasing cortisol levels. Indeed, cortisol hypersecretion has widely been used to define states of stress in human studies. Recently, hypocortisolism has

KARGER

Fax +41 61 306 12 34
E-Mail karger@karger.ch
www.karger.com

1021–7401/10/0173–0192$26.00/0

Accessible online at:
www.karger.com/nim

Dr. Moisés E. Bauer
Laboratory of Cellular and Molecular Immunology, Institute of Biomedical Research
PUCRS, Av. Ipiranga 6690, 2° andar, PO Box 1429
Porto Alegre, RS 90610-000 (Brazil)
Tel. +55 51 3320 3000, ext. 2725, Fax +55 51 3320 3312, E-Mail mebauer@pucrs.br

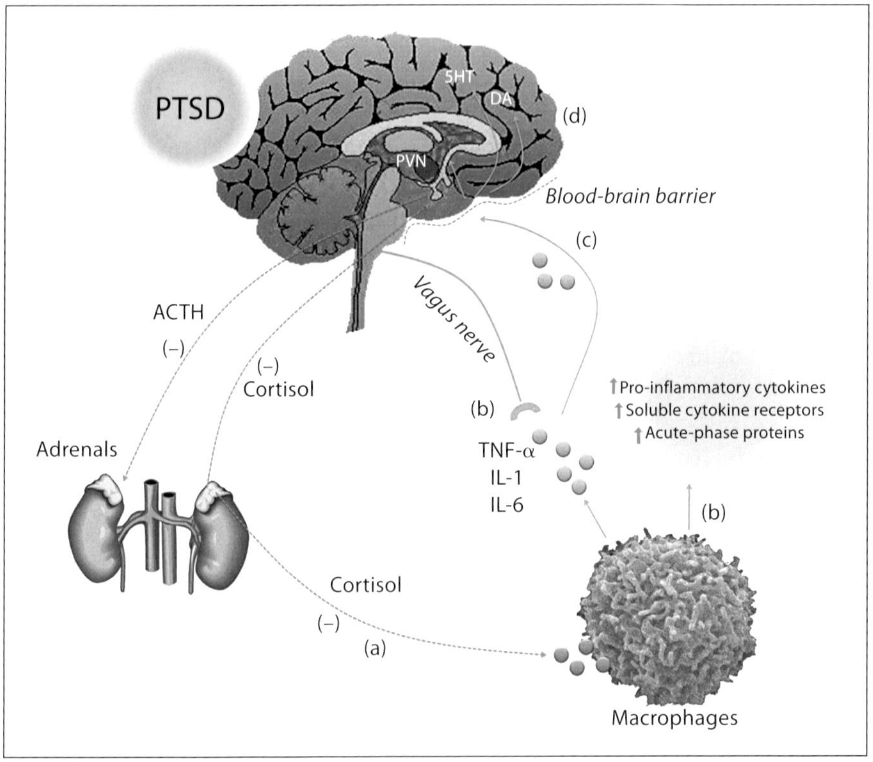

Color version available online

Fig. 1. Neuroimmune interactions during PTSD. Hypocortisolism is associated with lack of adequate control of the immune system (a), leading to low-grade inflammation as indicated by increased levels of pro-inflammatory cytokines (b). These cytokines, in turn, access the brain via afferent fibers (e.g. vagus nerve) (b) or through leaky regions of the blood-brain barrier (c) or through active transport molecules. Once in the brain (d), cytokine signals participate in pathways known to be involved in the development of depression, including: (1) altered metabolism of relevant neurotransmitters such as serotonin (5HT) and dopamine (DA), and (2) activation of CRH in the paraventricular nucleus (PVN) and the subsequent production and/or release of ACTH and glucocorticoids (cortisol).

also been observed in patients with burnout, physical complaints, chronic fatigue syndrome, fibromyalgia, chronic pelvic pain, asthma and others [1]. These data suggest that hypocortisolism is not a specific phenomenon of PTSD.

However, chronically elevated levels of cortisol seem to exist in children who are currently living in adverse situations. Studies performed with maltreated children or who are diagnosed with PTSD show hypercortisolemia [2]. Girls exposed to sexual abuse show an impaired HPA axis function following pharmacological or nonpharmacological challenge tests. In line with such results, Heim et al. [3] found that female adults with childhood sexual abuse had significantly higher cortisol and adrenocorticotropic hormone (ACTH) levels following exposure to acute psychosocial stress (Trier Social Stress Test, TSST) compared to controls. On the other hand, women with early childhood sexual abuse and PTSD had lower concentrations of cortisol during the afternoon hours (noon to 8 p.m.) compared with women with abuse without PTSD and women without abuse or PTSD [4]. It has been hypothesized that an early chronic increase of CRH would lead to downregulation of pituitary CRH receptors during life. This would be thus associated with adrenal insufficiency ('functional adrenalectomy'), and would ultimately explain the blunted cortisol levels found in women with a history of childhood abuse and PTSD.

Low-Grade Inflammation

The immune system is critically regulated by the glucocorticoids. In line with the lack of adequate glucocorticoid-mediated inhibition of immune responses, increasing evidence of immune activation has been reported in stress-related disorders characterized by hypocortisolism. There is growing evidence supporting the link between traumatic stress to a pro-inflammatory profile [5], with increasing serum concentrations of TNF-α, IFN-γ, IL-1β and IL-6. Recently, we observed that depressed patients with or without PTSD symptoms had higher soluble TNF receptor 2 levels in contrast to lower IL-2 and chemokine RANTES levels compared to healthy controls [6]. The low-grade inflammatory response has been linked to disease severity. PTSD patients seem to respond to mild everyday stressors with exaggerated anxiety responses that could potentially trigger the production of pro-inflammatory cytokines. It is also known that experimental psychosocial stress increase pro-inflammatory cytokines. The involvement of cytokines in the pathophysiology of PTSD may involve changes of synaptic transmission, especially in hippocampal-amygdala structures, influencing various aspects of memory related to trauma.

The phenomenon of low-grade inflammation could be also involved with increased morbidity in PTSD. Peripheral administration of pro-inflammatory cytokines or increased levels observed during infections has been associated with changes in the patient's behavior known as 'sickness behavior'. The patient becomes irritable and exhibits increased sleep, depression, fatigue, decreased appetite and sexual drive. Pro-inflammatory cytokines have been implicated in this phenomenon. One clinical example of the role of cytokines in determining behavioral changes comes from studies evaluating the biological effects of IFN-α. Depression has been reported in up to 60% of patients with hepatitis C under treatment with IFN-α. The HPA axis may also have its activity enhanced by pro-inflammatory cytokines; however, a positive relationship between increased HPA axis activity and markers of immune activation is not well established.

Increased Cell-Mediated Immunity and Activation Phenotype

In addition to low-grade inflammation, patients with PTSD also reported important changes in cell-mediated immunity. For instance, NK cells, lymphocytes, T cells have been found particularly increased [7]. The relative balance between Th1/Th2 immune responses seems to be balanced towards a potent Th1 immunity. Indeed, delayed-type hypersensitivity (DTH) was found enhanced in women with PTSD due to childhood sexual or physical abuse [8].

The phenotype of lymphocytes is also altered in PTSD, suggesting an activation profile. Increased counts of activated T ($CD2^+HLA^-DR^+$), B ($CD20^+CD23^+$) and NK ($CD16^+CD71^+$) cell subpopulations in women with PTSD due to war displacement have been reported [9]. Lymphocytes expressing the late ($CD71^+$) but not the early ($CD25^+$) activation marker were also elevated in displaced women. Another phenotype alteration is regarding the T cell memory profile, especially those associated with a history of childhood sexual abuse. An increased percentage of both central memory ($CD45RA^-CCR7^+$) and effector memory ($CD45RA^-CCR7^-$) T cell subsets has been observed in PTSD patients [10]. Interestingly, Sommershof et al. [10] also observed a ~50% drop of regulatory T cells ($CD4^+CD25^+FoxP3^+$) in PTSD patients as compared to healthy controls. This substantial decline of regulatory T cells (Tregs) could bear the risk of excessive inflammation due to suboptimum control of immune responses and provide further support to the pro-inflammatory profile observed in patients with PTSD. Therefore, PTSD patients could be at risk for inflammatory disorders. Indeed, deficiency or dysfunction of Tregs in humans has been linked to several inflammatory and auto-immune diseases including multiple sclerosis, asthma, type 1 diabetes, psoriasis, and rheumatoid arthritis.

Altered Peripheral Sensitivity to Glucocorticoids

The effects of glucocorticoids on the immune system are mediated via both intracellular and membrane-bound glucocorticoid receptors (GRs). However, the functional effect of a stress hormone will depend on the sensitivity of the target tissue for that particular hormone. A reliable way of assessing the cross talk between peripheral hormones and the immune system is to determine the functional hormone action in specific target cells. We have recently observed that dexamethasone (GR agonist) was less capable to suppress T cell proliferation of depressed women with long-standing PTSD symptoms due to childhood maltreatment, suggesting acquired steroid resistance. Conversely, it has also been shown that mononuclear cells from Bosnian war refugees with PTSD symptoms required less dexamethasone concentrations to inhibit cellular LPS-induced IL-6 and TNF-α secretion, suggesting increased sensitivity to glucocorticoids [11].

The magnitude of the biological effects of glucocorticoids is determined, among other factors, by the number and functionality of GRs. Yehuda et al. [12] reported increased densities of GR in peripheral lymphocytes of combat Vietnam veterans, without changes in cortisol levels. However, there are contradictory findings in the literature reporting lower GR densities with unaltered affinity for glucocorticoids. To what extent changes in glucocorticoid signaling in the immune system are related to fluctuations in cortisol levels or immune mediators (cytokines) remains to be determined.

Concluding Remarks

PTSD is associated with impaired homeostatic forces, leading to a significant allostatic load across the nervous, endocrine and immune systems. Hypocortisolism, impaired central and peripheral glucocorticoid signaling, low-grade inflammation and activation of cell-mediated immunity are commonly observed changes reported in PTSD. The constant stress experienced by PTSD patients may have important deleterious consequences and predispose the patient to stress-related disorders.

References

1 Raison CL, Miller AH: When not enough is too much: the role of insufficient glucocorticoid signaling in the pathophysiology of stress-related disorders. Am J Psychiatry 2003;160:1554–1565.

2 De Bellis MD: Abuse and ACTH response to corticotropin-releasing factor. Am J Psychiatry 2002;159:157; author reply 157–158.

3 Heim C, Newport DJ, Heit S, Graham YP, Wilcox M, Bonsall R, Miller AH, Nemeroff CB: Pituitary-adrenal and autonomic responses to stress in women after sexual and physical abuse in childhood. JAMA 2000; 284:592–597.

4 Bremner D, Vermetten E, Kelley ME: Cortisol, dehydroepiandrosterone, and estradiol measured over 24 hours in women with childhood sexual abuse-related posttraumatic stress disorder. J Nerv Ment Dis 2007; 195:919–927.

5 Hoge EA, Brandstetter K, Moshier S, Pollack MH, Wong KK, Simon NM: Broad spectrum of cytokine abnormalities in panic disorder and posttraumatic stress disorder. Depress Anxiety 2009;26:447–455.

6 Grassi-Oliveira R, Brietzke E, Pezzi JC, Lopes RP, Teixeira AL, Bauer ME: Increased soluble tumor necrosis factor-alpha receptors in patients with major depressive disorder. Psychiatry Clin Neurosci 2009;63:202–208.

7 Boscarino JA, Chang J: Higher abnormal leukocyte and lymphocyte counts 20 years after exposure to severe stress: research and clinical implications. Psychosom Med 1999; 61:378–386.

8 Altemus M, Cloitre M, Dhabhar FS: Enhanced cellular immune response in women with PTSD related to childhood abuse. Am J Psychiatry 2003;160:1705–1707.

9 Sabioncello A, Kocijan-Hercigonja D, Rabatic S, Tomasic J, Jeren T, Matijevic L, Rijavec M, Dekaris D: Immune, endocrine, and psychological responses in civilians displaced by war. Psychosom Med 2000;62:502–508.

10 Sommershof A, Aichinger H, Engler H, Adenauer H, Catani C, Boneberg EM, Elbert T, Groettrup M, Kolassa IT: Substantial reduction of naive and regulatory T cells following traumatic stress. Brain Behav Immun 2009;23:1117–1124.

11 Rohleder N, Joksimovic L, Wolf JM, Kirschbaum C: Hypocortisolism and increased glucocorticoid sensitivity of pro-inflammatory cytokine production in Bosnian war refugees with posttraumatic stress disorder. Biol Psychiatry 2004;55:745–751.

12 Yehuda R, Lowy MT, Southwick SM, Shaffer D, Giller EL Jr: Lymphocyte glucocorticoid receptor number in posttraumatic stress disorder. Am J Psychiatry 1991;148:499–504.

NeuroImmunoModulation

Neuroimmunomodulation 2010;17:196–199
DOI: 10.1159/000258722

Published online: February 4, 2010

Neuroimmune Interactions in Stress

Frederico A. Costa-Pinto João Palermo-Neto

Department of Pathology, Neuroimmunomodulation Research Group, School of Veterinary Medicine and Animal Science, University of São Paulo, São Paulo, Brazil

Key Words

Neuroimmunomodulation · Corticosterone · Hypothalamus-pituitary-adrenal axis · Psychoneuroimmunology

Abstract

Stress has long been recognized as a putative modulator of immunity. Several clinical and experimental reports point to a role of physical and psychological stressors on progression or resistance to disease. Nonetheless, literature in this field is sometimes controversial due to the wide variety of stressors employed and parameters of immunity analyzed. This variation should not be considered a consequence of methodological inaccuracy. The stress response, although theoretically stereotyped in nature, may lead to slightly different outcomes according to several modifiers. Our group has compared the effects of several stressors over different parameters of brain activity, behavior, immunity and glucocorticoid levels. These data show altogether that while increased turnover of noradrenaline in the hypothalamus, along with anxiety-like behaviors and increase in serum corticosterone are present very often, the magnitude of changes in immunity may vary considerably. Thus, we review data from our group generated over the past decade to support that effects of stressors on immunity and behavior highly depend on their specifics, animal model, frequency, duration, intensity, perception, and coping by the stressed animal.

Ever since its publication in a 1936 issue of *Nature*, Hans Selye's pioneer work 'A syndrome produced by diverse nocuous agents' became a cornerstone [1]. This brief, dense report tackled the effects of diverse, nonspecific nocuous stimuli (the *stressors*) on distinct physiological systems, constituting phases of a 'general adaptation syndrome'. Selye's work built the foundation for the study of the effects of stress and its associated hormones on brain function, behavior, and immunity, crucial to the establishment of what we now study in neuroimmunomodulation. The literature has then accumulated numerous reports ascribing effects on neuroimmune interactions during health and disease to several experimental stressors. The parameters analyzed include changes in brain activity, animal behavior, and immunity. An overwhelming amount of data has gathered from clinical reports and experimental studies and constituted unequivocal, but sometimes controversial, evidence that supports the biological relevance of stress-mediated neuroimmune interactions in health and disease.

Early studies in this area focused particularly on the suppressive effects of stress on immunity and collectively considered stressors as a single, homogeneous group, since their effects used to be considered stereotyped. Nonetheless, the past decades have witnessed the development of novel neuropsychiatry theories on stress and its role in neuroimmunomodulation. This new conceptual framework accounts for differences in stressors regarding their nature or origin (physical or psychological)

KARGER

Fax +41 61 306 12 34
E-Mail karger@karger.ch
www.karger.com

1021–7401/10/0173–0196$26.00/0

Accessible online at:
www.karger.com/nim

João Palermo-Neto
Av. Prof. Dr. Orlando M. de Paiva, 87
Cidade Universitária, São Paulo, SP 05508-270 (Brazil)
Tel. +55 11 3091 7685, Fax +55 11 3091 7829
E-Mail jpalermo@usp.br

Table 1. Compilation of results obtained with different stressors on brain activity and chemistry, animal behavior, immunity, and corticosterone levels

Stressor	Brain activity	Behavior	Immunity	Corticosterone	Reference
Inescapable footshock	↑ NA turnover in hypothalamus	anxiety in EPM	↓ macrophage activity and resistance to Ehrlich tumor	↑ plasma levels	2, 3
Watch footshock on cage mate	↑ NA turnover in hypothalamus	anxiety in EPM	↓ macrophage activity and resistance to Ehrlich tumor	↑ plasma levels	2
Prenatal footshock	↑ NA turnover in hypothalamus	anxiety in EPM	↓ macrophage activity	↑ plasma levels	4
Cohabitation with sick cage mate	↑ NA turnover in hypothalamus	↑ motor activity in OF	↓ neutrophil activity, ↓ DTH, ↓ differentiation of dendritic cells	baseline unchanged	5, 6
Individual housing	↑ NA turnover in hypothalamus	anxiety in EPM	↓ resistance to Ehrlich tumor	baseline unchanged but ↑ after immobilization	7
Social subordination	↑ NA turnover in hypothalamus	anxiety in EPM and OF	↓ neutrophil and NK cell activity; ↓ resistance to B16F10 metastases	baseline unchanged but ↑ after immobilization	8
Chemical stressors	↑ NA turnover and c-fos expression in hypothalamus	anxiety in EPM	↓ neutrophil and macrophage activity; ↓ resistance to infection	↑ plasma levels	9, 10

NA = Noradrenaline; EPM = elevated plus maze; OF = open field; DTH = delayed-type hypersensitivity; ↑ = increase; ↓ = decrease.

and temporal pattern (acute vs. chronic). Moreover, different parameters of immunity, innate and adaptive, have been assessed, adding complexity and variability to previous reports in the field. Altogether, stress assumed a more intricate position as a putative immunomodulator in a wide variety of biological responses. We review here a series of studies performed in our labs that employed specific stressors and their effects on neurochemistry, behavior and immunity (compiled in table 1). Our major goal is to bring attention to the necessity of dealing with the nature of stressors as variable, complex entities that may lead to differential neuroimmunological effects.

Employing semi-automated analysis of standard parameters of animal behavior such as motor activity and anxiety, in an open-field arena and in the elevated plus maze, respectively, we have focused on the effects of specific stressors on behavior and immunity. Palermo-Neto et al. [2] compared the effects of daily escapable or inescapable footshock stress for 6 days. The authors report increased levels of anxiety in the plus maze, associated with increased turnover of noradrenaline in the hypothalamus, increased serum levels of corticosterone, along with decreased activity of peritoneal macrophages and reduced resistance to the growth of the ascitic Ehrlich tumor. Stress effects on behavior and macrophage activity were not found following escapable footshocks, supporting that coping and manageability over the stressor may change its perception by the animal and therefore its effects [2]. Additionally, when inescapable footshock was associated with a rat model of experimental lung inflammation, the stressor exacerbated the effects of ovalbumin-induced asthma-like signals and increased the number of leukocytes in the bronchoalveolar lavage of allergic rats challenged with the antigen [3].

Prenatal stress has also been studied in the offspring of mice submitted to footshock during late pregnancy [4]. Juvenile mice from dams stressed during gestational days 15–19 displayed increased motor activity, particularly in the central open field, which suggests increased levels of anxiety-like behavior, even in the absence of altered exploration of the elevated plus maze [4]. Prenatal stress leads to decrease in spreading and phagocytosis by macrophages, along with reduction in nitric oxide secretion [4] and increased serum levels of corticosterone [unpubl.

results]. Interestingly, prenatally stressed mice respond differently when exposed to mild footshock stressors, similar to those applied to their mothers. While some parameters were unchanged in prenatally stressed exposed to postnatal footshock mice, some were attenuated, and others were enhanced [4].

Communication between conspecifics also plays a role in stress-induced immunomodulation. Mice watching their cage mates receiving footshock, which can be regarded as a natural psychological stressor, showed similar changes in brain function, behavior, and immunity as their companions [2]. Living with a sick cage mate, a putative rodent model for the *caregiver* situation in humans, also shed some light on the perception of sickness among conspecifics living in a dyad. Cohabitation with a tumor-bearing sick mate induced an increase in total motor activity, along with increased turnover of noradrenaline in the hypothalamus, but no changes in corticosterone [5, 6]. The companions of sick cage mates also have decreased neutrophil activity [5]. Cell-mediated immunity in these mice seems disturbed, with altered phenotype of dendritic cells. While spleen-derived Iab+CD11c+ cells show increased expression of CD80 costimulatory molecule, in vitro differentiation of these cells from bone marrow precursors in the presence of GM-CSF, IL-4 and LPS is partially blunted. Delayed-type hypersensivity to ovalbumin in these mice is deficient, associated with proliferation of a IL-10-secreting lymphocyte subpopulation [6].

Although sometimes still controversial, individual housing (IH) of rodents can lead to high levels of stress. After being housed in groups, mice were IH for 2 or 3 weeks. Corticosterone levels were similar in resting conditions, but peaked higher in IH animals following a single 30-min immobilization session. Additionally, IH mice spent less time in the open arms of an elevated plus maze, an indicative of higher anxiety levels. Moreover, when challenged with the Ehrlich tumor, these animals died slightly sooner than their counterparts, with higher number of tumor cells in their abdomens [7].

From an ethological standpoint, social stressors are extremely interesting and relevant since they tend to reproduce natural situations of life. The biology of dominant and subordinate mice has been focused in some studies from our group. In a stable hierarchy, subordinate mice display more anxiety-like behaviors in the open field and in the elevated plus maze, consistent with increased noradrenaline turnover in the hypothalamus. Furthermore, circulating neutrophils and NK cells from these mice showed decrease killing activity, when compared to cells obtained from their dominant cage mates. Transfer of B16F10 melanoma cells to subordinate mice lead to increased number of metastases in their lungs [8].

Chemically-induced stress has also been employed as a model of neuroimmune disturbance. Mice treated with picrotoxin, a noncompetitive $GABA_A$ receptor antagonist, have increased serum levels of corticosterone, higher turnover of noradrenaline in the hypothalamus, and increased anxiety in the elevated plus maze. Although not as drastic as the changes in immunity during physical stressors, picrotoxin induced a decrease in neutrophil activity [9]. Cyhalothrin, a synthetic type II pyrethroid insecticide, has also been used with a similar purpose by our group [10]. Treated rats display increased anxiety in the open field, increased c-fos expression and noradrenaline turnover in the hypothalamus, increased serum corticosterone levels, and reduced innate immunity [10] leading to diminished resistance to infection.

The balance between circulating levels of cytokines is crucial for regulating immune responses, and failure of this balance usually leads to disease. Since cytokines may have opposing effects in the brain, and their levels can be influenced by the brain directly or not, by adrenaline and glucocorticoids among other stress hormones, stressors may influence this delicate balance and change immunity.

Glucocorticoids seem a common link between the effects of stress on immunity, and in fact, many of the effects on circulating leukocytes described during stress may be ascribed to increased levels of this hormone. Several changes in immunity during stress are lacking in mice treated with methyrapone, reinforcing the role of glucocorticoids.

Nonetheless, there are cases in which immunity is altered during stress in the absence of altered corticosterone levels, pointing to a possible role of catecholamines. Additionally, stressors seem to strongly suppress Th1 adaptive immune responses, while skewing the balance towards a Th2 pattern of cytokine secretion. Glucocorticoids have long been shown to shift this balance, influencing the polarization of naïve T cells, possibly leading to decreased resistance to infections caused by several stressors, particularly in long-term or chronic conditions. However, not all stressors unbalance the Th1/Th2 (more recently Th1/Th17) equilibrium, hence their effects on adaptive immunity may vary, at least slightly.

Ongoing research in our labs focuses on the role of the sympathetic autonomic nervous system (SNAS) on the neuroimmune interactions during stress and also on the pathways and mechanisms that underlie the responses described here. We hope to find a complementary response in the SNAS during stress that would support the lack of participation of glucocorticoids in some cases. Also, the model of immune response employed and its parameters included for analysis may lead to different conclusions in regard to the effects of stress on immunity. We believe the body of evidence accumulated from studies performed by several groups, along with our own, supports that the neuroimmune consequences of stress vary according to several factors such as the nature of stressor, its magnitude and duration, onset, and degree of control over the stressor by the stressed animal.

References

1 Selye H: A syndrome produced by diverse nocuous agents: 1936. J Neuropsychiatry Clin Neurosci 1998;10:230–231.
2 Palermo-Neto J, de Oliveira Massoco C, Robespierre de Souza W: Effects of physical and psychological stressors on behavior, macrophage activity, and Ehrlich tumor growth. Brain Behav Immun 2003;17:43–54.
3 Portela C de P, Massoco C de O, de Lima WT, Palermo-Neto J: Stress-induced increment on total bronchoalveolar cell count in ova-sensitized rats. Physiol Behav 2001;72:415–420.
4 Fonseca ES, Massoco CO, Palermo-Neto J: Effects of prenatal stress on stress-induced changes in behavior and macrophage activity of mice. Physiol Behav 2002;77:205–215.
5 Alves GJ, Vismari L, Florio JC, Palermo-Neto J: Cohabitation with a sick cage mate: effects on noradrenaline turnover and neutrophil activity. Neurosci Res 2006;56:172–179.
6 Tomiyoshi MY, Sakai M, Baleeiro RB, Stankevicius D, Massoco CO, Palermo-Neto J, Barbuto JA: Cohabitation with a b16f10 melanoma-bearer cage mate influences behavior and dendritic cell phenotype in mice. Brain Behav Immun 2009;23:558–567.
7 Palermo-Neto J, Fonseca ES, Quinteiro-Filho WM, Correia CS, Sakai M: Effects of individual housing on behavior and resistance to Ehrlich tumor growth in mice. Physiol Behav 2008;95:435–440.
8 Sa-Rocha VM, Sa-Rocha LC, Palermo-Neto J: Variations in behavior, innate immunity and host resistance to b16f10 melanoma growth in mice that present social stable hierarchical ranks. Physiol Behav 2006;88:108–115.
9 Stankevicius D, Rodrigues-Costa EC, Camilo Florio J, Palermo-Neto J: Neuroendocrine, behavioral and macrophage activity changes induced by picrotoxin effects in mice. Neuropharmacology 2008;54:300–308.
10 Righi DA, Xavier FG, Palermo-Neto J: Effects of type II pyrethroid cyhalothrin on rat innate immunity: a flow cytometric study. Int Immunopharmacol 2009;9:148–152.

NeuroImmunoModulation

Neuroimmunomodulation 2010;17:200–201
DOI: 10.1159/000258723

Published online: February 4, 2010

Chronic Expression of Transforming Growth Factor-Beta Enhances Adult Neurogenesis

Patricia Mathieu[b] Ana Paula Piantanida[a] Fernando Pitossi[a]

[a]Institute Leloir Foundation, IIBBA-CONICET, [b]FFyB, UBA, Buenos Aires, Argentina

Key Words

Adult neurogenesis · Transforming growth factor-beta · Adenoviral vectors

Abstract

Neural stem cells reside in two neurogenic regions of the adult brain: the dentate gyrus of the hippocampus (DG) and the subventricular zone (SVZ). Their proliferation, differentiation, migration and survival are modulated by intrinsic and extrinsic signals, forming a neurogenic niche. Brain cytokines have only been recently regarded as possible components of this neurogenic niche. In particular, we have demonstrated that transforming growth factor-β (TGF-β) has a pro-neurogenic effect in the DG in a model of increased neurogenesis by adrenalectomy. We wanted to test whether TGF-β has a similar effect in another neurogenic region, namely the SVZ. To test this possibility, adult rats were injected with adenoviral vectors expressing TGF-β (Ad-TGF) or β-galactosidase (Ad-bgal) in the SVZ and neurogenesis was evaluated 3 weeks later. We have observed that chronic TGF-β expression increased neurogenesis in the ipsilateral hemisphere of Ad-TGF but not in Ad-bgal-treated rats compared to their contralateral side. In addition, an unspecific effect of the adenoviral vector per se could not be totally discarded. We conclude, under our experimental conditions, that TGF-β could enhance adult neurogenesis in the SVZ. This data increase the growing evidence supporting a pro-neurogenic role of anti-inflammatory cytokines in the adult brain.

In the adult mammal brain, there are certain neurogenic regions where neural stem/progenitor cells (NSC) proliferate and have the potential to differentiate into neurons, astrocytes and oligodendrocytes [1]. Adult neurogenesis is regulated by environmental signals collectively defined as the neurogenic niche. Several molecular components of the neurogenic niche have been identified including sonic hedgehog, bone morphogenic proteins, leukemia inhibitory factor and vascular endothelial growth factor [2]. Not only can brain cytokines mediate immune functions but they can also modulate several brain-associated processes independently of the immune system [3]. Only recently, it has been observed that pro-inflammatory cytokines such as IL-6 and IL-1 can diminish and anti-inflammatory cytokines such as transforming growth factor-β (TGF-β) and IL-4 can increment adult neurogenesis, respectively [4]. In particular, we have observed that TGF-β, an anti-inflammatory cytokine, has a positive effect on neurogenesis in the dentate gyrus of the adult hippocampus in a model of enhanced neurogenesis by adrenalectomy in vivo [5]. We wanted to explore the possibility that TGF-β could increase neurogenesis in another neurogenic area, the subventricular zone (SVZ) of the lateral ventricles.

To test this hypothesis, adult male Wistar rats (8–10 weeks old) were unilaterally injected with 1×10^7 particles of adenoviral vectors TGF-β (Ad-TGF) or β-galactosidase (Ad-bgal) as control, under ketamine chlorhydrate (80 mg/kg) and xylazine (8 mg/kg) anesthesia. This treatment allows transgenic expression for at least 14 days

KARGER

Fax +41 61 306 12 34
E-Mail karger@karger.ch
www.karger.com

1021–7401/10/0173–0200$26.00/0

Accessible online at:
www.karger.com/nim

Fernando Pitossi
Institute Leloir Foundation, IIBBA-CONICET
Patricias Argentinas 435
Buenos Aires (Argentina)
Tel. +54 11 5238 7500, Fax +54 11 5238 7501, E-Mail fpitossi@leloir.org.ar

in the brain ([6] and data not shown). The stereotaxic injections were performed with a 50-μm tipped fine glass capillary directed to the left SVZ at bregma, antero-posterior, +0.5 mm; lateral, +1.5 mm; ventral, –4.0 mm. One week after adenoviral injection, animals were injected intraperitoneally with 50 mg/kg/day of 5-bromo-2′-deoxyuridine (BrdU) during 7 days. Three weeks after adenoviral injection, animals were deeply anesthetized and perfused transcardially with heparinized saline and tissue was fixed with 4% paraformaldehyde in 0.1 M phosphate buffer (PB). Brains were removed and postfixed overnight at 4°C in 4% paraformaldehyde in PB, after which they were cryoprotected in 30% sucrose in PB and sliced coronally in 40-μm sections with a sliding cryostat. Animal procedures were performed according to the regulations for the use of laboratory animals of the National Institutes of Health, USA.

The amount of newly born neurons in the SVZ was determined by performing double immunofluorescence against BrdU (a marker of cell proliferation) and doublecortin (DCX, a marker of young neuronal phenotype) with specific antibodies. Briefly, one-in-six series of free-floating sections were incubated for 2 h in 50% formamide at 65°C, washed once in ×2 standard saline citrate (SSC; 0.3 M NaCl, 0.03 M sodium citrate), incubated for 30 min at 37°C in 2 N HCl, rinsed in 0.1 M borate buffer, pH 8.5, and thoroughly washed in Tris-buffered saline (TBS; Tris-HCl 50 mM pH 7.4, NaCl 150 mM). Sections were blocked in 0.1% Triton X-100, 1% donkey serum in TBS (blocking solution) for 40 min at room temperature (RT). Rat anti-BrdU (1:150; Abcam, UK) and rabbit anti-DCX (1:150; Abcam, UK) were diluted in blocking solution and sections were incubated for 72 h at 4°C. Sections were then incubated with Cy2-conjugated donkey anti-rat and Cy3-conjugated donkey anti-rabbit (1:200; Jackson Laboratories, West Grove, Pa., USA) for 2 h at room temperature (RT). Sections were mounted in Mowiol (Calbiochem, La Jolla, Calif., USA). Double-stained cells in the SVZ were quantified using z-scan confocal microscopy (Zeiss LSM 510 confocal-laser scanning microscope equipped with an argon and He/Ne laser that emitted at 488 and 568 nm, respectively) at ×20 magnification. Each cell was analysed along the entire 'z' axis. Between 200 and 600 BrdU-positive cells were counted to calculate double-labeled cell percentages, and the total number of double-labeled cells was estimated.

In the SVZ ipsilateral to the Ad-TGF injection, the number of newly born neurons was increased in comparison to the contralateral side (* $p < 0.05$; fig. 1). No similar effect was observed when the injected and uninjected SVZ of Ad-bgal-treated animals was compared (fig. 1). When the ipsilateral hemispheres of Ad-TGF and Ad-bgal-injected animals were analyzed, a tendency to an increase in neurogenesis was observed in the first group but it did not reach statistical significance (fig. 1), suggesting an effect of the adenoviral injection per se that precluded to draw conclusions from this comparison.

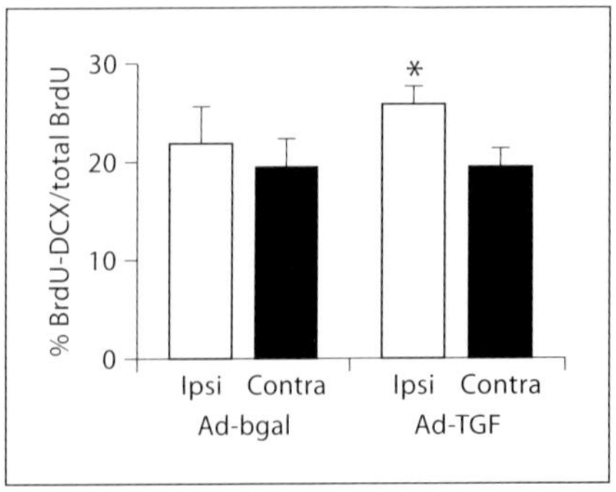

Fig. 1. Effect of TGF-β expression on neuronal differentiation in the SVZ. Quantification of the percentage of double-labeled cells in the SVZ among the BrdU-positive cell population in Ad-TGF-β and Ad-bgal-injected animals. Ad-TGF significantly increases the amount of BrdU/DCX-positive cells. Comparisons were performed using t test analysis (* $p < 0.05$). Values are the mean ± SEM. Ipsi = Ipsilateral; Contra = contralateral to adenoviral injection.

We conclude that chronic TGF-β expression could produce an increment in newborn neurons from the adult SVZ. A contribution of the adenoviral vector per se on this effect could not be discarded. These data support the idea of considering brain cytokines as part of the adult neurogenic niche. It also provides evidence in favor of considering anti-inflammatory cytokines as pro-neurogenic molecules in the adult brain.

References

1 Gage FH: Neurogenesis in the adult brain. J Neurosci 2002;22:612–613.
2 Alvarez-Buylla A, Lim DA: For the long run: maintaining germinal niches in the adult brain. Neuron 2004;41:683–686.
3 Besedovsky H: Immune-neuro-endocrine interactions: facts and hypotheses. Endocr Rev 1996;17:64–102.
4 Ekdahl CT, Kokaia Z, Lindvall O: Brain inflammation and adult neurogenesis: the dual role of microglia. Neuroscience 2009;158:1021–1029.
5 Battista D, et al: Neurogenic niche modulation by activated microglia: transforming growth factor beta increases neurogenesis in the adult dentate gyrus. Eur J Neurosci 2006;23:83–93.
6 Ferrari CC, et al: Progressive neurodegeneration and motor disabilities induced by chronic expression of IL-1beta in the substantia nigra. Neurobiol Dis 2006;24:183–193.

NeuroImmunoModulation

Neuroimmunomodulation 2010;17:202–204
DOI: 10.1159/000258724

Published online: February 4, 2010

Neuroimmunomodulation in the Pathogenesis of Alzheimer's Disease

Inelia Morales Gonzalo Farías Ricardo B. Maccioni

Laboratory of Cellular and Molecular Neurosciences (LCMN), Faculty of Sciences and International Center for Biomedicine (ICC), Ñuñoa Santiago, Chile

Key Words

Neuroinflammation · Microglia cells · Cellular signaling · Neuroprotection · Alzheimer's disease

Abstract

Evidence has been cumulated on the role of microglia cells deregulation and alterations in their interaction patterns with brain neurons, in the pathway towards neurodegeneration in Alzheimer's disease (AD). After the failure of the amyloid hypothesis to explain AD pathogenesis, current hypotheses focus on tau self-polymerization into pathological oligomers and filaments as a major culprit for neurofibrillary degeneration. It is worth pointing out that formation of tau polymers is consistent with the clinical and neuropathological observations, and that tangles are pathognomonic of AD and related tau disorders. In this context, inflammatory processes play a major role in neuronal degeneration. On the basis of studies on microglia and neuronal cultures, together with experiments in animal models, and the clinical evidence, we postulated that a series of endogenous damage signals activate microglia cells, inducing NFκ-β with the consequent release of cytokine mediators such as TNF-α, IL-6 and IL-1β. An overexpression of these mediators may trigger signaling cascades in neurons leading to activation of protein kinases gsk3β, cdk5, abl kinases, along with inactivation of phosphatases such as PP1, with the resulting hyperphosphorylation and self-aggregation of tau protein into neurotoxic oligomeric species.

Introduction

Increasing evidence has been cumulated that neuroimmune networks contribute to the maintenance of neurogenesis [1]. The microglia (brain immune cells) and neuronal cells are directly involved in this process. Under normal physiological conditions, cytokines and chemokines are involved in brain repair and recovery. Cross talk between inflammatory mediators and neural stem cells appears to be critical for neural development. In addition, microglia supports neural stem cell renewal, migration and lineage specification. Precise control of proliferation and differentiation of multipotent stem cells is crucial for the development of the central nervous system (CNS) as well as for adult brain repair [2]. However, deregulation of the cross talks between microglia and neuronal cells occurs upon overactivation of microglia cells [3]. We postulated that this overactivation (fig. 1) appears to be a result of multiple damage signals, e.g. iron overload, oxidative stress molecules, β-amyloid (Aβ) oligomers, low-density lipoprotein components of human plasma, ischemia, brain trauma, etc. [4, 5]. These factors promote erroneous signaling cascades in microglia cells, via RAGE, toll-like receptor 4 (TLR4) and several other glial receptors, thus inducing proinflammatory cytokine production. Cytokines and chemokines are important neuroinflammatory mediators, whose overexpression results from these damage signals that trigger Alzheimer's disease (AD) [6].

KARGER

Fax +41 61 306 12 34
E-Mail karger@karger.ch
www.karger.com

1021–7401/10/0173–0202$26.00/0

Accessible online at:
www.karger.com/nim

Prof. Dr. R.B. Maccioni
LCMN, Edificio Milenio
Las Encinas 3370
Ñuñoa Santiago (Chile)
Tel. +56 2 978 7228, E-Mail rmaccion@manquehue.net

Alzheimer's Disease Is a Disorder of the Innate Immune System

Microglia cells are normally beneficial for brain function. Helpful actions include phagocytosis and killing pathogens. However, when overactive (fig. 1), they have harmful actions including excess production of oxygen free radicals, complement proteins, inflammatory cytokines, prostaglandins, glutamate and many as yet unidentified products. We postulate that the major driving force in AD is neuroinflammation, by activation of the innate immune system. In this context, AD is an autotoxic disorder. This type of disorders affects mainly the elderly, as a difference from autoimmune diseases that involve the adaptive immune system and strike the young. In this context, a series of danger signals, as indicated above, trigger the inflammatory cascade. Considering the foregoing, we have postulated the neuroimmunomodulation hypothesis for AD pathogenesis, which integrates the triggering factors with innate immunity response, and their effects on neuronal cells [6]. Proinflammatory cytokines signal through different neuronal receptors, thus activating protein kinases involved in tau hyperphosphorylation – like cdk5 and its activator p35 – with the subsequent tau modifications, conformational changes and initiation of the self-aggregation process [5, 6]. Self-polymerized tau oligomers appear as a neurotoxic agent in the pathway toward neuronal degeneration. This hypothesis is supported by cellular and molecular evidence [7] as well as by extensive clinical data indicating that long treatments with anti-inflammatory drugs reduce the risk of AD [8]. Moreover, studies in our laboratory with activated rat microglia cells in primary cultures showed that cytokine-containing conditioned media from these cells promote degeneration, as well as tau hyperphosphorylation, of cultured hippocampal neurons obtained from rat embryos.

Among microglial receptors tagged by damage signals are the innate immune receptor TLR4, a pattern recognition receptor. Its function within the CNS has been recently expanded as new data suggests its influence on microglia activity. TLR4 is expressed primarily on microglia, where it can affect neurons upon activation and subsequent cytokine production. Its expression and signaling activities vary widely under pathological conditions, as evidenced in studies of ischemic stroke, AD and neuropathic pain. This receptor is known for its capacity to detect lipopolysaccharide (LPS), and it responds to endogenous signals of cellular damage. Damage signals such as Aβ but also opioids have recently been reported

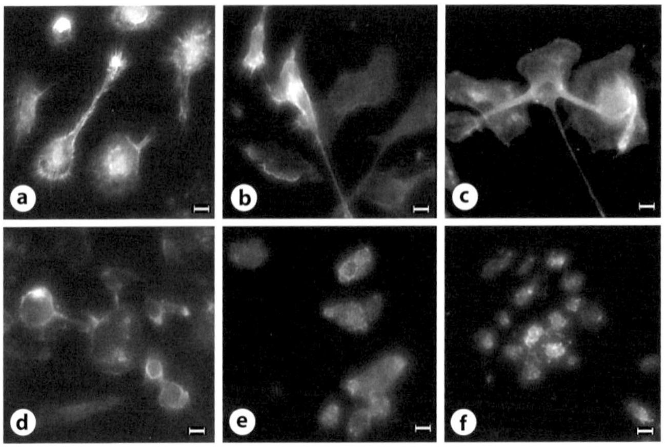

Fig. 1. Activation of microglia cells in primary culture by ascending concentrations of hydrogen peroxide and LPS. **a** = Control, **b–e** = 1, 10, 100, 400 μM H_2O_2, **f** = 1 μg/ml LPS. Immunofluorescence with anti-isolectin antibody specific for microglia and faloidin which specifically tag the actin cytoskeleton. A modification in cellular morphology, in which microglia cells turn from a resting, branched morphology to an amoeboid state, can clearly be appreciated in relation to activation after exposure to noxic stimuli. Bars = 5 μm.

to induce TLR4 signaling. This protein has been crystallized, providing clues on its mechanism of action. These exciting discoveries have highlighted the new functional aspects on TLR4 signaling [9], thus facilitating potential transfer of this knowledge into drug developments for AD and other brain disorders.

Microglial Activation and Anomalous Neuronal Signaling Cascades

Microglia cells are the representatives of the immune system in the CNS, and thus are related to immune response and homeostasis. These cells may remain inactivated for long periods of time, and suddenly change their behavior due to its high sensitivity for various signals from their brain environment. When a physiological or pathological stimulus is sensed, cells are capable of migrating to the area of injury, become activated and phagocytic brain macrophages, representing a system of defense and neuroprotection. This transformation is regulated and accompanied by diverse cytokines (mostly proinflammatory) and cytotoxic molecules (free radicals of oxygen, nitric oxide, complement factors, etc.) that allow communication with other inactivated microglia, and with brain and immune system cells. On the other hand, neurons respond to activated microglia cells with different types of signals.

Pathologies such as AD and other related degenerative brain disorders appear to arise when the damage signals inducing microglia cell activation act in a sustained fashion over long periods of time [6], causing the overactivation of microglia (fig. 1) and the excessive secretion of pro-inflammatory cytokines and cytotoxic molecules that finally leads to damage in brain tissue.

Thus, a series of innate damage signals that would be involved in detonating the activation of microglia have been described [5]. These signals include AGES, HMBG1, S-100 proteins, Aβ peptide oligomers (but not the fibrillar aggregates), which activate microglia via RAGE receptor. Furthermore, oxidized low-density lipoprotein activates the TLRs receptors, particularly TLR4, thus inducing activation. Other signs of damage such as mechanical damage and damage caused by oxyradicals also induce the production of Aβ oligomers, AGE and S-100 protein, which contributes to the process of microglial activation [5].

All these signs of damage trigger alarm mechanisms in the innate immune system, resulting in microglial activation, starting with an increase in the activity of the transcription factor NFκ-β, which in turn induces an increased production of the cytokines TNF-α, IL-6 and IL-1β [for details, refer to ref. 5]. Excessive release of these cytokines results in a local inflammatory response and neuronal degradation.

In neuronal cells, the effects of TNF-α have not been associated with any particular phenomenon of neuroprotection, but an effect of this cytokine in decreasing the activity of cdk5, under specific cell conditions, has been observed. Furthermore, IL-6 induces hyperphosphorylation of tau protein by interfering in the regulation of cdk5/p35 complex by increasing the intraneuronal concentration of cdk5. IL-6 also activates the JAK/STATs and MAPK-p38 systems [10]. IL-6 role in neuroinflammation and neurodegeneration has also been associated with an effect on cognitive impairment.

IL-1β is also involved in regulating the cdk5/p35 complex, and also induces the production of nitric oxide in the hippocampal neuronal cells, which is closely related to cell death [3].

Therefore, the effects of microglia overactivation can be summarized in the excessive release of pro-inflammatory cytokines, which generate changes in the intraneuronal regulation, most of which converge in the alteration of tau protein. These alterations lead to profound changes in the neuronal dynamics and metabolism and subsequent cell death. As a result of deregulation of neuron-microglia cross-talks, neurons also respond to restore regulatory patterns, until the inflammatory driving force results in neuronal degeneration.

Acknowledgements

Research has been supported by grant RG-081-91219 from the Alzheimer's Association, USA, and Fondecyt 1080254.

References

1 Kempermann G, Chesler EJ, Lu L, Williams RW, Gage FH: Natural variation and genetic covariance in adult hippocampal neurogenesis. Proc Natl Acad Sci USA 2006;103:780–785.

2 Battista D, Ferrari CC, Gage FH, Pitossi FJ: Neurogenic niche modulation by activated microglia: transforming growth factor beta increases neurogenesis in the adult dentate gyrus. Eur J Neurosci 2006;23:83–93.

3 Rojo L, Fernández J, Maccioni AA, Jimenez J, Maccioni RB: Neuroinflammation: implications for pathogenesis and molecular diagnosis of Alzheimer's disease. Arch Med Res 2008;39:1–16.

4 Lavados M, Guillón M, Mujica C, Rojo L, Fuentes P, Maccioni RB: Mild cognitive impairment and Alzheimer patients display different levels of Redox-active CSF iron. J Alzheimer's Dis 2008;13:225–232.

5 Fernandez J, Rojo L, Kuljis R, Maccioni RB: The damage signals hypothesis of Alzheimer's disease pathogenesis. J Alzheimer's Dis 2008;14:329–333.

6 Maccioni RB, Fernandez J, Rojo L, Kuljis R: Neuroimmunomodulation in Alzheimer's disease. Ann NY Acad Sci 2008;1153:240–247.

7 Orellana D, Quintanilla R, Maccioni RB: Neuroprotective effect of TNF alpha against the beta-amyloid neurotoxicity mediated by CDK5 kinase. Biochim Biophys Acta 2007; 1773:254–263.

8 McGeer PL, Schulzer M, McGeer EG: Arthritis and anti inflammatory agents as possible protective factors for Alzheimer's disease: a review of 17 epidemiologic studies. Neurology 1996;47:425–432.

9 Covacu R, Arvidsson L, Andersson A, Khademi M, Erlandsson-Harris H, Harris RA, Svensson MA, Olsson T, Brundin L: TLR activation induces TNF-alpha production from adult neural stem/progenitor cells. J Immunol 2009;182:6889–6895.

10 Quintanilla R, Orellana D, Gonzalez-Billault C, Maccioni RB: Interleukin-6 induces Alzheimer's phosphorylation of tau protein by deregulating the cdk5/p35 pathway. Exp Cell Res 2004;295:245–257.

NeuroImmunoModulation

Neuroimmunomodulation 2010;17:205–208
DOI: 10.1159/000258725

Published online: February 4, 2010

Evaluation of Stress Systems by Applying Noninvasive Methodologies: Measurements of Neuroimmune Biomarkers in the Sweat, Heart Rate Variability and Salivary Cortisol

Andrea H. Marques Marni N. Silverman Esther M. Sternberg

National Institute of Mental Health/NIH, Rockville, Md., USA

Key Words

Cytokines · Neuropeptides · Cardiovascular system · HPA axis

Abstract

The two main arms of the stress system include the autonomic nervous system (ANS) and the hypothalamic-pituitary-adrenal (HPA) axis. These two neural stress systems coordinate the response of many other physiological systems to a stressor, including the immune and cardiovascular systems, bringing the body back to homeostasis. The nervous and immune systems communicate with each other in a bidirectional manner. In this review, we will discuss the use of noninvasive methods to evaluate the immune system, ANS and HPA axis. Collection of sweat and saliva, and measurement of heart rate variability are noninvasive methods that can be applied to evaluate neuroimmune interactions. Recently, we validated a new methodology to simultaneously evaluate a large array of neural and immune biomarkers in sweat, collected through cutaneous sweat patches and measured by recycling immunoaffinity chromatography. Noninvasive and ambulatory methodologies of biomarker collection can overcome several limitations intrinsic to invasive methods, such as reducing the stress triggered by collection itself and allowing a wider application to field and community-based settings. Ultimately, simultaneous evaluation of neural and immune systems with noninvasive techniques will help elucidate the underlying interactions of these systems and their role in disease susceptibility and progression of stress-related disorders.

Introduction

Two main pathways by which psychological stress is relayed to the body are the hypothalamic-pituitary-adrenal (HPA) axis (neuroendocrine route, resultant release of glucocorticoids – cortisol) and the sympathetic nervous system (SNS, neural route, resultant release of catecholamines – noradrenaline/adrenaline – and neuropeptides). Dysregulation of either of these stress systems can lead to dysregulation of multiple other physiological systems, including the immune and cardiovascular systems, metabolic function and behavior, leading to a maladaptive response to stress (fig. 1).

The nervous and immune systems communicate with each other in a bidirectional manner [1, 2]. Indeed, dysregulation of neural-immune interactions are described

KARGER

Fax +41 61 306 12 34
E-Mail karger@karger.ch
www.karger.com

Accessible online at:
www.karger.com/nim

Esther M. Sternberg, MD, Integrative Neural Immune Program and Chief
Section on Neuroendocrine Immunology and Behavior National Institute of
Mental Health/NIH, 5625 Fishers Lane MSC 9401, Rm. 4N-13B
Rockville, MD 20892-9401 (USA)
Tel. +1 301 402 2773, Fax +1 301 496 6095, E-Mail sternbee@mail.nih.gov

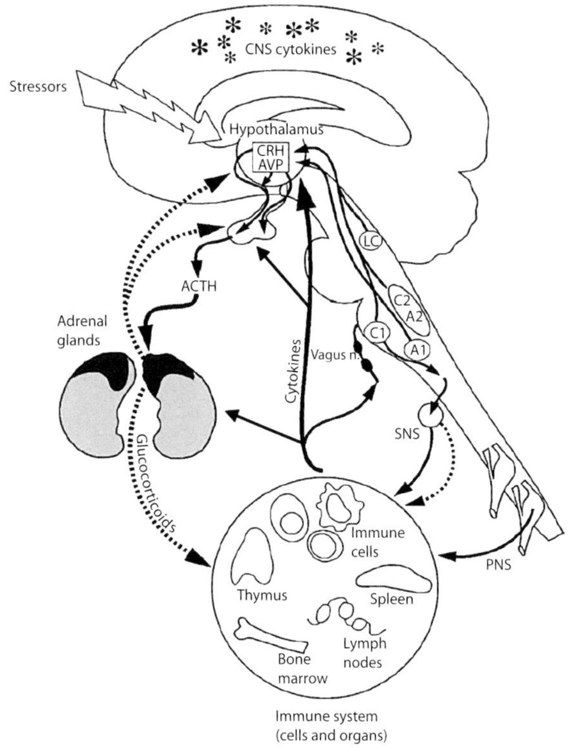

Fig. 1. Diagram of the routes of communication between the brain and immune system, including the HPA axis, autonomic nervous system, and cytokine interactions with both of these systems. CNS = Central nervous system; SNS = sympathetic nervous system; PNS = peripheral nervous system; CRH = corticotropin-releasing hormone; AVP = arginine vasopressin; ACTH = adrenocorticotropic hormone. Reprinted with modifications by permission from Webster et al. [9].

in many stress-related disorders including inflammatory, autoimmune, metabolic and cardiovascular disease, as well as psychiatric disorders. Simultaneous evaluation of stress and immune systems with noninvasive, and thus non-stress-inducing, techniques will help to elucidate the underlying interactions of these systems and their role in disease susceptibility and progression of stress-related disorders. In this review, we will briefly discuss noninvasive methodologies that can be simultaneously applied in order to evaluate neural and immune system biomarkers in sweat, the ANS by measuring heart rate variability (HRV) and the HPA axis by measuring cortisol in saliva.

Neuroimmune Biomarker Evaluation

One noninvasive and nonstressful approach to evaluating neural and immune systems is through collection of sweat. We have validated a methodology to simultaneously evaluate a large array of neural and immune biomarkers in sweat, collected through cutaneous sweat patches.

The cutaneous sweat patch is commercially available and FDA approved. It is easily applied at any time of day and can be worn for an extended period of time with minimal discomfort. In addition, since sweat collection is over a 24-hour period, rather than a single time point, the use of the sweat patch may overcome circadian variability exhibited by analytes of interest. In our validation study, subjects were instructed to apply two sweat patches at 8 a.m. on the day before coming into the laboratory for blood collection, and wore them for 24 h. On the next day, blood samples were obtained at 8 a.m., after an overnight fast, prior to the removal of the sweat patches. The sweat patch was placed in a zip lock bag and stored at –70 °C until time of biomarker analysis. This simple procedure had high rates of compliance for proper self-application of the sweat patch [3]. After collection, plasma and sweat neuroimmune biomarkers were detected by recycling immunoaffinity chromatography (RIC) coupled with laser-induced fluorescence at the National Institute of Biomedical Imaging and Bioengineering. This methodology has been used to measure cytokines in plasma and cervical secretions [4], in cord blood and postnatal serum from newborns and more recently in sweat and plasma of healthy premenopausal women and women with depression [3, 5]. Briefly, sweat analytes are vacuum-extracted from the patch, protein content is normalized before applying the extract to an immunoaffinity column array system [4] and results are verified by mass spectrometry and MALDI-TOF. RIC is a single-antibody system that uses a set of high-performance liquid chromatographic immunoaffinity columns in series, with each column immunospecific for a targeted, fluorescently labeled analyte [4]. The advantage of this methodology is that it is highly sensitive and specific and allows measurements of a much larger number of analytes per unit of fluid than are detectable with others methods. In addition, minute volumes of fluid can be analyzed (e.g. a specimen volume of only 25 μl is required). One disadvantage of the RIC technology is that it is labor-intensive and therefore not easily applicable in a clinical lab setting. Studies are ongoing to validate other more clinically accessible, high-throughput and sensitive methodologies for analyte quantification.

In our initial validation studies, we showed that immune biomarkers, such as pro-inflammatory cytokines, in sweat were tightly correlated with plasma levels in healthy controls [3]. These results were obtained using RIC and linear regression analysis, which confirmed that sweat levels were highly predictive of plasma levels. In addition, our preliminary data in a population of women with major depressive disorder (MDD) show elevated sweat levels of pro-inflammatory cytokines, sympathetic neuropeptides (neuropeptide-Y [NPY]) and pain-related neuropeptides (substance P [SP], calcitonin gene-related peptide [CGRP]), but decreased parasympathetic (vasoactive intestinal peptide [VIP]) neuropeptides relative to controls, which strongly correlated with plasma levels [5]. This pattern is consistent with a shift in MDD from parasympathetic to sympathetic tone and an underlying pro-inflammatory state that could account for enhanced susceptibility to conditions known to be comorbidly expressed with MDD, including cardiovascular disease, osteoporosis and diabetes. Moreover, biomarker levels strongly correlated with symptoms of depression and anxiety, indicating functional significance of these biomarker profiles.

Neural Pathway Evaluation: Peripheral Nervous System and Autonomic Nervous System

The neural stress system consists of the peripheral nervous system and the ANS. Both systems play an important role in the stress response and modulate the immune system at local and regional levels. The peripheral nervous system regulates the immune system at sites of inflammation through the release of neuropeptides that tend to be pro-inflammatory [2]. As mentioned above, a noninvasive method to measure neuropeptides is through collection of sweat. Our previous studies showed that neuropeptides, such as NPY, VIP, SP and CGRP, can be measured in sweat and are tightly correlated with levels in plasma in patients with history of depression [5]. The sympathetic and parasympathetic (vagus nerve, mediated by acetylcholine) branches of the ANS play an important role in the regulation of the cardiovascular system and the immune system [6, 7], where the parasympathetic nervous system has been shown to have an anti-inflammatory influence on the immune system [7].

Evaluation of the ANS can also be performed noninvasively through measurement of HRV. HRV is a term that describes variations of both instantaneous heart rate and the interval between consecutive beats. A prominent circadian variation in HRV, with significant increases during the night and decreases during the day, is observed in healthy individuals. Previous studies have shown that this increase in nighttime HRV is blunted by acute stress, as well as conditions such as chronic alcoholism [6]. Decreased HRV, indicative of reduced parasympathetic/vagal tone, is an independent risk factor for morbidity and mortality.

HPA Axis Evaluation

Salivary cortisol is an easily obtainable biofluid and noninvasive source for evaluating the HPA axis. This methodology has been widely applied in field-related research settings through the development of adequate ambulatory technology to collect saliva. However, it is important to emphasize that the use of this technique has its limitation and the analysis of the data has to take into account the research question. Studies have shown that measuring cortisol after awakening – the 'cortisol awakening response' (CAR) – is considered an indicator of basal HPA axis activity. In addition, CAR is influenced by several factors such as age, gender, stress perception, health status and lifestyle behaviors. In addition, recent studies have shown that several daily measurements are necessary to assess the CAR [8].

Conclusion

Simultaneous and repeated evaluation of stress-related systems with noninvasive techniques can help elucidate the underlying interactions of the immune system, ANS, and HPA axis, and their role in disease susceptibility and progression of stress-related disorders. We have established a methodology to simultaneously evaluate a large array of neural and immune biomarkers in sweat, collected through commercially available, FDA-approved cutaneous sweat patches. Applying this new methodology together with two already established methods, HRV to evaluate the ANS and salivary cortisol measurements to evaluate the HPA axis, can aid in identifying biomarker patterns associated with disease stage, severity and outcome, as well as treatment efficacy.

Sweat and saliva collection overcome several of the limitations intrinsic to blood collection. These sampling approaches represent a minimally invasive technique, without pain or distress, for measuring neuroimmune and endocrine parameters, respectively.

Ultimately, these noninvasive methodologies could provide a 'molecular signature' for clinical subtypes within a heterogeneous disorder, to be used for diagnostic and prognostic purposes; to allow for earlier intervention in asymptomatic conditions; for optimization of individualized treatment regimens; for patient monitoring in remote areas and in large-scale epidemiological settings; for monitoring patients in which invasive methodologies are unfeasible; and to shed light on mechanisms that underly individual vulnerability or resilience to development of stress-related diseases/disorders.

References

1 Silverman MN, et al: Immune modulation of the hypothalamic-pituitary-adrenal (HPA) axis during viral infection. Viral Immunol 2005;18:41–78.
2 Sternberg EM: Neural regulation of innate immunity: a coordinated nonspecific host response to pathogens. Nat Rev Immunol 2006;6:318–328.
3 Marques-Deak A, et al: Measurement of cytokines in sweat patches and plasma in healthy women: validation in a controlled study. J Immunol Methods 2006;315:99–109.
4 Phillips TM: Multi-analyte analysis of biological fluids with a recycling immunoaffinity column array. J Biochem Biophys Methods 2001;49:253–262.
5 Cizza G, et al: Elevated neuroimmune biomarkers in sweat patches and plasma of premenopausal women with major depressive disorder in remission: the POWER study. Biol Psychiatry 2008;64:907–911.
6 Thayer JF: Vagal tone and the inflammatory reflex. Cleve Clin J Med 2009;76(suppl 2):S23–S26.
7 Tracey KJ: Physiology and immunology of the cholinergic anti-inflammatory pathway. J Clin Invest 2007;117:289–296.
8 Fries EL, Dettenborn J, Kirschbaum C: The cortisol awakening response (CAR): facts and future directions. Int J Psychophysiol 2009;72:67–73.
9 Webster JI, Tonelli L, Sternberg EM: Neuroendocrine regulation of immunity. Annu Rev Immunol 2002;20:125–163.

NeuroImmunoModulation

Neuroimmunomodulation 2010;17:209–212
DOI: 10.1159/000258726

Published online: February 4, 2010

Stress in Wildlife Species: Noninvasive Monitoring of Glucocorticoids

Marta C. Romano[a] Alba Zulema Rodas[a, b] Ricardo A. Valdez[a]
Sandra Elizabeth Hernández[b] Francisco Galindo[b] Domingo Canales[c]
Dulce Maria Brousset[b]

[a]Departamento de Fisiología, Biofísica y Neurociencias, CINVESTAV-IPN, [b]Departamento de Etología, Fauna Silvestre y Animales de Laboratorio, Facultad de Medicina Veterinaria y Zootecnia, Universidad Nacional Autónoma de México, y [c]Instituto de Neuroetología, Universidad Veracruzana, Xalapa, México

Key Words
Cortisol · Noninvasive techniques · Wildlife species

Abstract
Depression and stress are related pathologies extensively studied in humans. However, this relationship is not well known in animals kept in zoos and even less known in wild animals. In zoo animals, acute and chronic stress caused by difficulties in coping with stressors such as public presence and noise, among others, can induce the appearance of repetitive pathological behaviors such as stereotypies, many times associated with organic pathologies that deeply affect their health and welfare. In the wild, factors such as deforestation, habitat fragmentation, lack of food and water, and human disturbances are potential causes of acute and chronic stress for the resident fauna. Glucocorticoids (GC) have been extensively used as stress indicators in many species including humans. Since chase and handling of wild animals immediately raise their GC serum levels, noninvasive methods have been developed to assess stress without interference caused by sample collection. The hormones and their metabolites can be measured in various body fluids and excreta and detect basal feedback free hormone concentrations as well as the response to ACTH and handling. In order to study the influence of disturbing factors we have measured GC as stress indicators by noninvasive techniques in dolphins and felids (ocelots, jaguarundis and margays) and cortisol and testosterone in spider monkeys.

Introduction

Depression and stress are related pathologies extensively studied in humans; however, this relationship is not well understood in wild animals kept at zoos and even less known in animals living in the wild. Acute and chronic stress in zoo animals, caused by difficulties in coping with stressors as public presence, noise, lack of space and natural substrate, among others, can induce the appearance of repetitive pathological behaviors such as stereotypies or apathy, many times associated to organic pathologies that deeply affect their health and welfare. In the wild, factors such as deforestation, habitat fragmentation, deficient food and water resources, or human disturbances are potential causes of acute and chronic stress for the resident fauna. Glucocorticoids

KARGER
Fax +41 61 306 12 34
E-Mail karger@karger.ch
www.karger.com

1021–7401/10/0173–0209$26.00/0

Accessible online at:
www.karger.com/nim

Dr. M.C. Romano
Departamento de Fisiología, Biofísica y Neurociencias, CINVESTAV-IPN
Apdo Postal 14-740, México DF 0700 (México)
Tel. +52 55 5061 3961, Fax +52 55 5061 3800, ext. 5109
E-Mail mromano@fisio.cinvestav.mx

(GC) have been extensively used as stress indicators in many species including the human. Since chase and handling of wild animals immediately raise GC serum levels, noninvasive methods have been developed to evaluate stress without interference caused by sample collection. The hormones and their metabolites can be measured in various body fluids and excreta and the technique detects baseline feedback free hormone concentrations, as well as the response to ACTH, handling, anesthesia or other stressors [1–4].

We include here examples of studies made by our group on the use of noninvasive techniques to evaluate the influence of disturbing factors in captive dolphins, wild felids (ocelot, jaguarundis and margays) and spider monkeys. An extensive revision of this theme is behind the permitted extension of this paper and should be found elsewhere in the related literature. As can be appreciated, the information provided by cortisol data was enriched when parallel studies of behavior were performed. Complementary data, as the animal clinical story that provides information on health, reproduction, etc., are extremely useful; this multidisciplinary approach gives a better understanding of animal welfare and how they cope with stressful conditions.

Saliva Glucocorticoid Measurements: The Case of Dolphins

Because of their small molecular weight and lipid solubility, GC passes quickly from serum to saliva, where can be directly measured by radioimmunoassay (RIA). They represent approximately 10% of GC serum concentration. This noninvasive technique was described years ago by Walker et al. [5] and can be used in trained animals and humans, even in newborns. We have investigated if cortisol was present in dolphin's saliva. We used the technique to evaluate stress in captive dolphins *(Tursiops truncatus)* trained to open their mouth voluntarily; the technique allowed daily saliva collection for 1 month. Cortisol was directly assayed in the samples by RIA and values were compared to serum ones obtained in parallel. Simultaneous behavioral observations were used to detect the association between GC concentration and stressful conditions [6]. This paper is one example of the usefulness of techniques that permit long-term sampling without opening doors to microbe invasion as can occur in repetitive skin punctures.

Behavior and Fecal Cortisol as Noninvasive Indicators to Assess Environmental Manipulations on Captive Ocelots *(Leopardus pardalis)*, Margays *(Leopardus wiedii)* and Jaguarundis *(Herpailurus yaguarondi)*

These three endangered felid species are native to Mexico, but there is little interest to exhibit them because the low activity and stereotypic pacing these animals present in captivity. The lack of space and natural substrate in zoos and the regular predictable food schedule can alter the motivation of behavior affecting their welfare. In order to improve it, a study was conducted to evaluate the effects of environmental enrichment programs, comparing the behavior and fecal cortisol levels of six ocelots, seven margays and six jaguarundis kept in three different zoos. The study compressed three periods of observation and sampling: 1 week previous (P1), 1 week during environmental enrichment manipulations (P2), and 1 week after (P3). Here we only show the cortisol results corresponding to the P1 group. Videotapes were used to obtain information on behavior repertory, individual time budget, social interactions and abnormalities (data not shown here). At the same time, fecal samples were collected daily to evaluate cortisol levels. Fecal samples were kept frozen and analyzed by RIA using an extraction protocol described by Brown and Wildt [1] and modified by Brousset [7] using a commercial cortisol assay (Coat-A-Count, DPCl solid phase); the intra- and inter-variation coefficient assays were <10% and all the results are expressed on dry matter.

The average (mean ± SD) fecal cortisol levels were different between species, being higher in jaguarundis (2,696 ± 2,123 ng/g dry feces), than in ocelots (1,561 ± 1,514 ng/g dry feces) and margays (870 ± 77 ng/g dry feces) ($p < 0.05$). This difference could be explained by a family characteristic since high fecal cortisol concentrations were also found in puma's feces, a species closely related to the jaguarundi. Other possibilities could be a difference in cortisol excretion pathways or a different response to stressors. Jaguarundis, as well as the animals on exhibiting enclosures and those that were pets previous to being housed at the zoo, had statistically significant higher fecal cortisol values.

Another study evaluated the impact of translocation into new enclosures in a couple of ocelots. The results showed that there is a relation between fecal cortisol and arousal and exploring behaviors. There is a positive statistically significant correlation between fecal cortisol and arousal behaviors, indicating that the increase in the

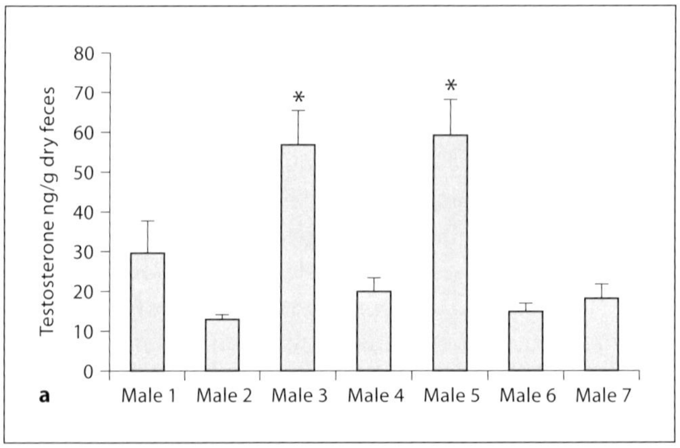

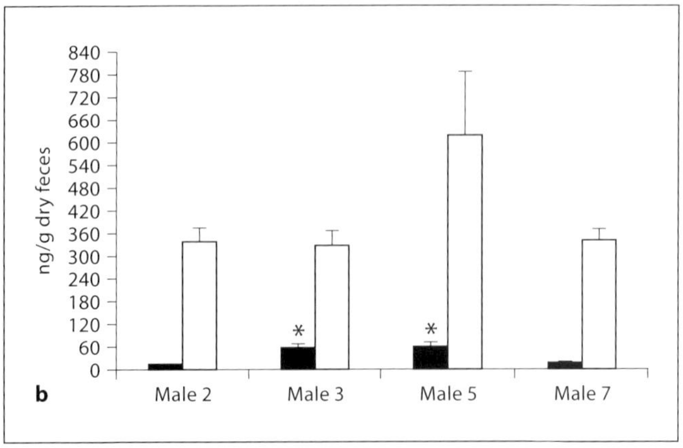

Fig. 1. Mean fecal testosterone and cortisol in spider monkeys *(Ateles geoffroyi)*. **a** Mean fecal testosterone of seven spider monkeys. The animals were sampled once a week for 3 months. Data show mean ± SE (males 1, 2, 3, 4 and 6, n = 12; males 5 and 7, n = 13). * $p < 0.05$. **b** Mean fecal testosterone and cortisol concentration of four spider monkeys. The animals were sampled as described in **a**. Testosterone (black bars) and cortisol (white bars) were measured in the same samples by radioimmunoassay. Data show mean ± SE (males 2 and 3, n = 12; males 5 and 7, n = 13). * $p < 0.05$.

frequency of this behavior is significantly associated with the increase of cortisol concentration. This higher adrenal activity could be related to an alarm response as a result of being exposed to new stimuli at the new enclosure. On the other hand, there is a negative statistically significant correlation between exploring behaviors and cortisol levels; increases in exploring behaviors were related to low levels of cortisol which suggests that living in environments that make these behaviors possible ameliorates stress in these animals. Therefore, this noninvasive technique, together with behavioral observations, is a useful tool to investigate if a zoo animal is coping adequately with a new environment.

Primates: Glucocorticoids and Steroid Reproductive Hormones in the Spider Monkey

Primates as many other species are threaten by environmental perturbations as forest fragmentation and habitat destruction, and are also exposed to being hunted. These stressful situations have a physiological cost and cause health problems such as alteration in growth and reproduction, immune system inhibition and even depression that is conducive to several infectious diseases. The synthesis and excretion of GC by Old World monkeys have been investigated in the last century [2]. However, interest on hormones related to stress in New World monkeys is relatively recent. Three of these species live in forests in Mexico: *Ateles geoffroyi*, *Alouatta pigra* and *Alouatta palliata*. All of them are endangered by environmental perturbations of their habitats and even hunting. On the other hand, serum testosterone concentration has been shown to correlate with aggressive behavior in many species [11].

Noninvasive techniques are useful to study stress and reproduction in free-living and captive primate populations. Using these techniques, the effect of stressful situations like forest fragmentation in the habitat of *Alouatta pigra* monkeys [8], or how a group of *Alouatta palliata* species solve stressful problems created for example by the arrival of a new male to a resident group [9] have been published. Influences on fecal cortisol of environmental conditions such as forest conservation have been recently reported in free-living Yucatan spider monkeys [10].

We have also evaluated the fecal cortisol and testosterone concentration in a group of spider monkeys *(Ateles geoffroyi)* living in special facilities designed by the Universidad Veracruzana at Catemaco, Veracruz, Mexico (Parque de la Flora y Fauna Silvestre Tropical). The animals have been confiscated from illegal hunters. For testosterone determinations, the study group comprised 7 adult males: male 1 (6 years), male 2 (8 years), male 3 (15 years), male 4 (16 years), male 5 (16 years), male 6 (21 years) and male 7 (21 years). Feces were collected once a week at 7 a.m. for a period of 1 year, but only those obtained in the first 3 months were evaluated for this preliminary study. For simultaneous cortisol and testosterone determinations, only data from 4 of the 7 monkeys are shown here.

The samples were kept frozen until extracted and analyzed by RIA using the protocol for cortisol determination developed by Brown and Wildt [1] and modified by Brousset [7] described above, and ^{125}I-CORT-CT2 CIS Bio Internacional® kits were used for cortisol determination. Ether extracted fecal samples were used to detect testosterone by RIA using ^{3}H-testosterone (1,2,6,7-^{3}H (N); Perkin Elmer Life Sciences Inc.®) as the tracer. Results are expressed as ng/g dry matter.

Figure 1a shows the mean ± SE of fecal testosterone concentration of males sampled for three months. Note that monkeys 3 and 5 have significantly higher testosterone concentrations compared with the rest of the group; to our knowledge, this is the first report on fecal testosterone concentration in spider monkeys. Behavioral observations showed that these monkeys were the most aggressive of the group. Figure 1b shows the mean ± SE fecal testosterone and cortisol concentrations obtained after 3 months of sampling.

Therefore, the data exposed here show that noninvasive techniques are useful to follow the hormone excretion of wild free and captive animals for long periods, thereby avoiding harm by repeated manipulations involving anesthesia or at least sedation for blood sampling. Manipulation and anesthesia increased cortisol levels within minutes; thereby, data obtained under these conditions cannot be considered as baseline. On the contrary, noninvasive techniques such as the ones used in the present studies represent baseline conditions. Therefore, any observed cortisol change is the result of behavioral, reproductive or social events not related to the sampling itself.

References

1 Brown JL, Wildt DE: Assessing reproductive status in wild felids by non-invasive faecal steroid monitoring. Int Zoo Yb 1997;35:173–191.
2 Wasser SK, Hunt KE, Brown JL, Cooper K, Crockett CM, Bechert U, Millspaugh JJ, Larson S, Monfort SL: A generalized fecal glucocorticoid assay for use in a diverse array of nondomestic mammalian and avian species. Endocrinology 2000;120:260–275.
3 Touma C, Palme R: Measuring fecal glucocorticoid metabolites in mammals and birds: the importance of validation. Ann NY Acad Sci 2005;1046:54–74.
4 Graham LH: Non-invasive monitoring of reproduction in zoo and wildlife species. Ann Rev Biomed Sci 2004;6:91–98.
5 Walker RF, Riad-Fahmy D, Read GF: Adrenal status assessed by direct radioimmunoassay of cortisol in whole saliva or parathyroid saliva. Clin Chem 1978;24:1460–1463.
6 Pedernera-Romano C, Valdez RA, Singh S, Chiappa X, Romano MC, Galindo F: Salivary cortisol in captive dolphins (*Tursiops truncatus*): a non-invasive technique. Anim Welfare 2006;15:359–362.
7 Brousset DM: Efecto del enriquecimiento ambiental sobre el bienestar de tres especies de felinos mexicanos en peligro de extinción (ocelote, margay y jaguarundi) mantenidos en cautiverio; Tesis de Doctorado, FMVZ-UNAM, 2003.
8 Martínez-Mota R, Valdespino C, Sánchez-Ramos MA, Serio-Silva JC: Effects of forest fragmentation on the physiological stress response of black howler monkeys. Anim Conserv 2007;10:374–379.
9 Cristobal-Azkarate J, Chavaira R, Boeck L, Rodríguez-Luna E, Vea J: Glucocorticoid levels in free ranging resident mantled howlers: a study of coping strategies. Am J Primatol 2007;69:1–11.
10 Rangel-Negrin A, Alfaro JL, Valdez RA, Romano MC, Serio-Silva JC: Stress in Yucatan spider monkeys: effects of environmental conditions on fecal cortisol levels in wild and captive populations. Anim Conserv 2009: 1–9.
11 Linch JW, Ziegler TE, Strier KB: Individual and seasonal variation in fecal testosterone and cortisol levels of wild male tufted capuchin monkeys, *Cebus paella nigritus*. Horm Behav 2002;41:275–287.

NeuroImmunoModulation

Neuroimmunomodulation 2010;17:213–216
DOI: 10.1159/000258727

Published online: February 4, 2010

Models of Aging of Neuroimmunomodulation: Strategies for Its Improvement

Mónica De la Fuente[a] Lydia Gimenez-Llort[b]

[a]Department of Physiology (Animal Physiology II), Faculty of Biology, Complutense University of Madrid, Madrid, and [b]Department of Psychiatry and Forensic Medicine, Institut de Neurosciències, Universitat Autònoma de Barcelona, Bellaterra, Spain

Key Words
Immunosenescence · Premature aging · Enriched environments

Abstract
Communication between the nervous and the immune systems suffers impairment with aging, which explains the altered homeostasis and the resulting increase of morbidity and mortality in aged subjects. In humans, rats and specially in mice, we have proposed several models to study this fact. The established models of premature aging have been mice and humans with poor response to stress and anxiety versus subjects of the same chronological age without that characteristic, isolation, males versus females, menopausal models (in rodents after ovariectomy) and obesity. In all cases, the prematurely aged animals suffer an alteration of the nervous system (shown by behavioral tests) and immunosenescence as well as oxidative and inflammatory stress, which is followed by early mortality. In addition, in the above-mentioned models and in normal chronological aging, we have observed the effect of several lifestyle strategies, such as ingestion of adequate amounts of antioxidants, performance of moderate physical exercise, and different kinds of environmental enrichment, which improve the function of the immune cells and their redox state as well as animal behavior. Therefore, they retard the aging process and seem to increase the longevity of the individuals.

Aging Process, Biological Age Concept and Longevity

The universal process of aging may be defined as a progressive and general decrease of organism functions that leads to a lower ability to adaptively react to changes and preserve homeostasis. This accumulation of adverse changes with the passing of time, although they should not be considered a disease, strongly increases the risk of disease and finally results in death. However, the aging process is very heterogeneous and, thus, there are different rates of physiological changes in the various systems of the organism and in the diverse members of a population of the same chronological age. This justifies the introduction of the concept of 'biological aging', which determines the level of aging experienced by each individual and therefore his life expectancy. Thus, biological age is related to mean longevity, which can be defined as the mean of the time that the members of a population that have been born on the same date live. Subjects of a population with a higher rate of aging show an older biological age and a shorter life span.

Although many single-cause theories have been proposed to explain the aging process, an integrated theory of aging has also been recently published [1]. In answer to the question 'how' does aging happen, we propose that the aging process is a chronic oxidative stress condition (increase of oxidant compounds and decrease of antioxi-

KARGER

Fax +41 61 306 12 34
E-Mail karger@karger.ch
www.karger.com

1021–7401/10/0173–0213$26.00/0

Accessible online at:
www.karger.com/nim

Prof. Mónica De la Fuente, PhD
Department of Physiology (Animal Physiology II), Faculty of Biology
Complutense University of Madrid
José Antonio Novais 2, ES–28040 Madrid (Spain)
Tel. +34 91 394 4989, Fax +34 91 394 4935, E-Mail mondelaf@bio.ucm.es

dant defenses), which is linked to many age-related changes that affect a large number of parameters including morphology, physiology and behavior, at all levels of organization: molecular, cellular, tissue, organic and that of the whole individual. In addition, since emerging evidence shows a close link between oxidation and inflammation, and with aging the pro-inflammatory compounds increase to levels higher than those of the anti-inflammatory compounds, leading to inflammatory stress, an oxi-inflamm-aging has been proposed as the cause of the loss of function that appears with senescence [1].

Neuroendocrine-Immune Communication in Aging: Role of the Immune System in Loss of Homeostasis of Aging

With aging there is an impairment of the physiological systems in which the regulatory systems, namely the nervous, endocrine and immune systems, are the most affected as well as neuroendocrine-immune communication. Moreover, we have to realize that aging of the immune and neuroendocrine systems are interdependent processes [2]. Thus, age-related alterations of the regulatory systems lead to loss of homeostasis and therefore to the increase in morbidity and mortality that appears with age [1, 3] (fig. 1). Although the proposed concept of homeorrhesis, which refers to the fact that the set point of homeostasis changes during the different phases of life, including aging [2], is acceptable, it is evident that the level of homeostasis established in aged subjects is not very appropriate to confirm adequate functions. In fact, only aged individuals that maintain functional parameters healthy at the levels of adults reach very high longevity [1].

In addition, age-related changes are linked to chronic oxidative and inflammatory stress affecting all cells of the organism and specially those of the regulatory systems, which explains their impaired function [3]. Moreover, the immune system, due to its capacity of producing oxidant and inflammatory compounds in order to eliminate foreign agents, could be involved with the rate of aging if its age-related oxidative and inflammatory stress is not controlled. Thus, the changes in the immune system with age, denominated immunosenescence, could accelerate aging of the organism. In this context, a relation between the redox and inflammatory state of the immune cells, their functional capacities and the life span of the subjects has been proposed [1, 3] (fig. 1). In fact, human centenarians show levels of oxidative stress and function similar to those in adults (30-year-old) and lower oxidative stress and better function than those found in 70-year-old subjects in their immune cells [4]. Similar finding have been obtained on very long-lived mice [5].

Models for the Study of Aging of Neuroimmunomodulation

Support for the above-mentioned hypotheses may be obtained by the study of animal models in which subjects have an altered nervous system, with abnormal behavior parameters, immunosenescence as well as a great oxidative and inflammatory stress in its immune cells, and decreased longevity. In this context, we have investigated the following models (fig. 1):

Models of Poor Response to Stress, Anxiety and Depression in Mice and Humans

We have established a model of premature aging in mice based on altered stress-related behavioral response and immunosenescence [6]. The premature aging mice (PAM) show, with respect to non-PAM (NPAM) of the same chronological age, an impaired behavioral response with increased levels of anxiety, deficient immune function, oxidative stress and decreased life span [6]. A model of depression in mice has been proposed based on isolation of females in old age. These animals show altered behavior, immunosenescence and oxidative stress. Moreover, human subjects with stress-related disorders and suffering from anxiety or depression show a significant immunosenescence and oxidative stress [7].

Males versus Females

In mammalian species, females have a longer mean life span than males, which seems to be an effect of their less oxidized condition, in part due to the estrogens. Thus, we have observed this different life expectancy both in rats and mice, and that immune functions are better in females than males. Moreover, the redox state of female leukocytes is better than that of males [1, 8].

Menopausal Models

Menopausal women as well as ovariectomized rats and mice (a good model for mimicking human menopause) show premature immunosenescence and high oxidative stress situation [1, 8, 9]. This premature aging model in mice is also confirmed by alterations of several behavior parameters [unpubl. data].

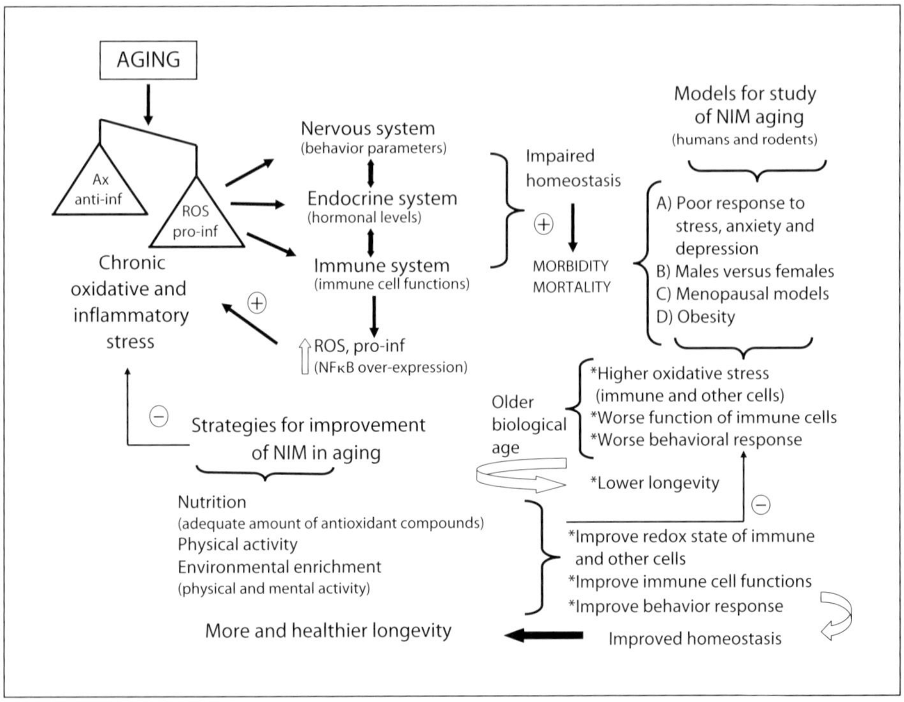

Fig. 1. Aging is a chronic oxidative stress condition affecting all cells, especially those of the regulatory systems, i.e. the nervous, endocrine and immune system, and the communication among them. This explains the impaired homeostasis and the increased morbidity and mortality found in old age. In humans and rodents we have proposed several models for the study of aging of neuroimmunomodulation (NIM). Animals with poor response to stress, anxiety and depression, males versus females, females with menopause/ovariectomy, and subjects with obesity show high oxidative stress in the immune and other cells, and impaired immune cell functions and behavioral responses. Thus, they have an older biological age and consequently show lower longevity. Several lifestyle strategies, such as adequate ingestion of antioxidant compounds, the performance of physical activity and appropriate environmental enrichment, improve immune functions, redox state and behavioral responses. Thus, they retard the aging process, improving homeostasis and increasing the longevity of the individuals. Ax = Antioxidant compounds; anti-inf = anti-inflammatory compounds; ROS = reactive oxygen species; pro-inf = pro-inflammatory compounds.

Obesity Models

Obese subjects, compared to nonobese subjects of the same chronological age, show worse immune functions and high oxidation-inflammation stress, which have been observed in both genetically and diet-induced obese rats [1].

Strategies for the Improvement of Neuroimmunomodulation in Aging

The oxidation-inflammation theory of aging is supported by work on the above-mentioned different models. Moreover, the basis of the age-related deterioration of the homeostatic systems and their communication is the chronic oxidative stress, and this is increased more or less depending, in part, on the degree of control of oxidation and inflammation of the immune system of each subject, which is related to the function capacity of its immune cells [1]. Therefore, it is convenient to test the effects of strategies based on improving several lifestyle environmental factors to retard the aging process, analyzing immune cell functions and their redox state. Further, the study of behavior parameters could give a more convincing confirmation of the proposed theory (fig. 1).

Role of a Diet Enriched with Antioxidants

In experimental animals and human subjects, the ingestion of a diet enriched with adequate amounts of antioxidants has been shown to be useful for maintaining an optimum redox balance, decreasing oxidative stress in immune cells and improving their function. Moreover, in mice, the ingestion of antioxidant improves the nervous function and consequently the behavior response. Since these effects are similar in mice and humans and because these changes in mice are accompanied by an increase in life span, it is probable that a similar effect could be obtained in humans [1, 3, 9]. We have also observed these effects in the mice anxiety model of PAM [6].

Role of Physical Activity

A moderate physical activity improves immune cell function and the redox state in both humans and rodents. Moreover, a moderate amount of physical exercise increases the level of antioxidant defenses in the immune cells [10].

Role of Environmental Enrichment

Enriched environments by intellectual and/or physical activities have been found to slow down many adverse effects of aging. Two different kinds of environmental enrichment have been used on mice to study their effect on behavior, immune cell functions, oxidation state and longevity. One of the environmental enrichments consisted of diverse objects of different shapes and colors (changed every 2 days) placed in the cages. The animals submitted to this strategy of lifestyle show an improvement in behavior parameters, immune functions and redox state. Moreover, their longevity was increased. A new environmental enrichment strategy for improvement in behavior, immune cell functions and redox state in mice has been hydrotherapy (bath for 15 min, 5 days a week for 2 or 4 weeks) (fig. 1).

Conclusions

There are several animal models for studying the aging of neuroimmunomodulation and confirming the role of the immune system in oxi-inflamm-aging. In these models, the subjects with worse behavior responses, immune functions and redox state show premature aging and early mortality. Several lifestyle strategies such as a better nutrition with adequate amounts of antioxidant compounds, mental and physical activity, and social relations seems useful to improve nervous and immune functions as well as the redox state and therefore retard the unavoidable aging process and increase the longevity of those subjects (fig. 1).

Support

MCINN (BFU2008-04336); Research Group UCM (910379); RETICEF (RD06/0013/0003).

References

1 De la Fuente M, Miquel J: An update of the oxidation-Inflammation theory of aging: the involvement of the immune system in oxi-inflamm-aging. Curr Pharm Design 2009;15:3003–3026.
2 Goya RG: The immune-neuroendocrine homeostatic network and aging. Gerontology 1991;37:208–213.
3 De la Fuente M: Role of neuroimmunomodulation in aging. Neuroimmunomodulation 2008;15:213–223.
4 Alonso-Fernandez P, Puerto M, Maté I, Ribera JM, De la Fuente M: Neutrophils of centenarians show function levels similar to those of young adults. J Am Geriatr Soc 2008;56:2244–2251.
5 Puerto M, Guayerbas N, Alvarez P, De la Fuente M: Modulation of neuropeptide Y and norepinephrine on several leucocyte functions in adult, old and very old mice. J Neuroimmunol 2005;165:33–40.
6 Viveros MP, Arranz L, Hernanz A, Miquel J, De la Fuente M: A model of premature ageing in mice based on altered stress-related behavioural response and immunosenescence. Neuroimmunomodulation 2007; 14: 157–162.
7 Arranz L, De Vicente A, Muñoz M, De la Fuente M: Impairment immune function in a homeless population with stress-related disorders. Neuroimmunomodulation 2009; 16:251–260.
8 De la Fuente M, Baeza I, Guayerbas N, Puerto M, Castillo C, Salazar V, Ariznavarreta C, F-Tresguerres JA: Changes with aging in several leukocyte functions of male and female rats. Biogerontology 2004;5:389–400.
9 Arranz L, Fernandez C, Rodriguez A, Ribera JM, De la Fuente M: The glutathione precursor N-acetylcysteine improves immune function in postmenopausal women. Free Rad Biol Med 2008;45:1252–1262.
10 De la Fuente M, Hernanz A, Vallejo MC: The immune system in the oxidation stress conditions of aging and hypertension: favorable effects of antioxidants and physical exercise. Antioxidants Redox Signals 2005;7:1356–1366.

NeuroImmunoModulation

Neuroimmunomodulation 2010;17:217–220
DOI: 10.1159/000258728

Published online: February 4, 2010

The CXCL12/CXCR4 Pair in Aged Human Thymus

Carmen Hernández-López[a] Alberto Varas[b] Rosa Sacedón[b] Victor G. Martínez[b] Laura Hidalgo[b] Jaris Valencia[b] Agustín G. Zapata[c] Ángeles Vicente[b]

[a]Center for Cytometry and Microscopy, [b]Department of Cell Biology, School of Medicine, and [c]Faculty of Biology, Complutense University of Madrid, Madrid, Spain

Key Words
Chemokines · CXCL12/CXCR4 · Human thymus · Aging · T cell maturation

Abstract
CXCL12 is an important CXC chemokine involved in numerous biological processes. We had previously demonstrated the synergistic participation of CXCL12 and IL-7 in the control of both survival and proliferation of $CD34^+$ human thymic lymphoid progenitors. On this basis, we hypothesize a presumptive role for CXCL12 and its receptor, CXCR4, in the thymus involution. In this respect, in the current report we describe the expression of both molecules in the human thymus during aging. Our results demonstrate that, despite the profound alterations observed in the thymic epithelial microenvironment of aged thymuses, the proportions of different CD4/CD8 thymocyte subsets do not undergo significant variations. Remarkably, a strong CXCL12 expression was found in older thymuses, which appeared in the same locations as in younger thymuses: the subcapsulary and medullary areas. The proportions of $CXCR4^+$ cells, most of them belonging to the $CD3^-$ compartment, showed no important variations in the older thymuses. However, within the $CD34^+$ cell population, a significant reduction in the expression of CXCR4 molecules was observed.

Introduction

Chemokines are small, soluble proteins (about 10 kDa) capable to produce a chemotactic cellular response. The chemokine family, which approximately comprises 50 members and 25 receptors, has been divided into four groups based on the position of the four conserved cysteine residues in the N-terminal region. With a few exceptions, CC chemokines bind to CC receptors, whereas CXC chemokines activate CXC receptors. Chemokine receptors belong to the family of G-protein-coupled receptors that activate adenylate-cyclase, phospholipases, GTPases (Rho, Rac, Cdc42) and major kinases (MAPK, PI3K) [1].

CXCL12 is an important member of the CXC subfamily that was firstly isolated from a murine bone marrow stroma cell line and has pleiotropic effects on the lympho-hematopoietic system as well as on the nervous system. CXCL12 was initially reported as a highly effective chemoattractant for lymphocytes and monocytes but not for neutrophils. Later it was recognized for regulating mature T and B lymphocyte survival and the generation of memory T cells [2]. In addition, CXCL12 and its receptor CXCR4 are key factors to regulate homing/mobilization of hematopoietic stem cells between bone marrow and peripheral blood, a process that undergoes catecholamine-mediated circadian variations [3]. On the

KARGER

Fax +41 61 306 12 34
E-Mail karger@karger.ch
www.karger.com

1021–7401/10/0173–0217$26.00/0

Accessible online at:
www.karger.com/nim

Carmen Hernández-López
Center for Cytometry and Microscopy
Complutense University of Madrid
ES–28040 Madrid (Spain)
Tel. +34 913 944 938, Fax +34 913 944 191, E-Mail carmenh@bio.ucm.es

other hand, CXCL12 and CXCR4 are constitutively expressed in the central nervous system and modulate neurotransmission, neurotoxicity and neuroglial interactions [1].

The involvement of CXCL12/CXCR4 in T cell differentiation is controversial. Although studies on CXCL12/CXCR4 gene disrupted mice suggested that these molecules are not required for the generation of a normal murine T cell population, other studies pointed out a role for CXCL12 in T cell differentiation. Several years ago, we demonstrated that CXCL12/CXCR4 signaling is not critical for the $CD34^+$ precursor cell recruitment to the human thymus but CXCL12 participates in the control of human lymphoid precursor cell survival and proliferation [4]. In this process, CXCL12 acts synergistically with IL-7, but not with other cytokines such as SCF (stem cell factor) or Flt3L (FMS-like tyrosine kinase 3 ligand), known to be important for the biology of lymphoid progenitors. IL-7 upregulates the CXCR4 expression on $CD34^+$ human lymphoid progenitors and, at the same time, stimulates the CXCL12 production by thymic epithelial cells (TEC). In turn, CXCL12 downregulates the IL-7 production by TEC.

The capacity of CXCL12 for controlling survival of thymic cells is not restricted to the thymocyte lineage. We recently demonstrated that human thymic dendritic cells (DC) express CXCR4 and produce CXCL12 that increases the survival and allostimulatory capacities of DC [5].

Based on these previous results, we hypothesize that since CXCL12 affects viability and proliferation of $CD34^+$ progenitor cells and their effects are related with IL-7/IL-7R signaling reported to be involved in thymus involution, this chemokine could be important to recover the thymus from physiological or experimentally induced conditions that course with decreased thymocyte production. Therefore, the current results are devoted to the analysis of CXCL12/CXCR4 condition in the involuted thymus that occurs during human aging.

Morphological Changes in the Human Thymus during Aging

The first signs of histological involution were clearly evidenced in 15- to 20-year-old human thymuses, markedly increasing in 30- to 40-year-old samples. Thymic involution coursed with disappearance of a clear cortex-medulla demarcation, principally due to extreme reduction of the cortical area that, in some older samples, appeared reduced to small groups of $CD1^+$ cells. Accordingly, the medullary area was proportionally increased but also appeared importantly altered. Other authors have described similar features in the involuted thymuses during aging, including significant reduction of the thymic surface area, decline of MHC class II and keratin expression and increased presence on certain molecules, such as Notch1 and Delta [6]. The condition of thymic medulla during aging is controversial. Some authors have described fewer changes in the medulla than in the thymic cortex of aged thymuses, but others suggest a parallel decline of both thymic compartments [6]. Retraction of epithelial cell processes in all thymic compartments also occurred in the older thymuses, a feature that has been related with the appearance of epithelial-free areas in the involuted thymuses [6].

Slight Changes in the Proportions of CD4/CD8 Thymocyte Subsets Occur in Aged Human Thymus

Despite the described profound alterations occurring in the thymic epithelial microenvironment of aged thymus, no significant variations were observed in the proportions of the different thymocyte subsets defined by the expression of CD4/CD8 markers. Analysis of human samples from postnatal to 70-year-old thymuses showed just a slight increase in the older ones in the proportions of DN and SP (both $CD4^+CD8^-$ and $CD4^-CD8^+$) cells. Correspondingly, decreased proportions of DP thymocytes occurred in those older thymuses that could be related with an increased percentage of apoptotic DP cells described in those thymuses [7].

CXCL12 Production in Older Human Thymuses

CXCL12 was expressed in the older thymuses in the same locations than in the younger ones [4]. By using specific markers for cortical and medullary TEC in combination with antibodies against CXCL12 we observed that CXCL12 expression occurred in the subcapsulary cortical area and in both the $TE\text{-}4^+$ TEC and Hassall's bodies of thymic medulla (fig. 1a). It is important to remark that, since thymus size decreases during aging, the relative area occupied by $CXCL12^+$ cells is presumably larger in older thymuses than in younger ones.

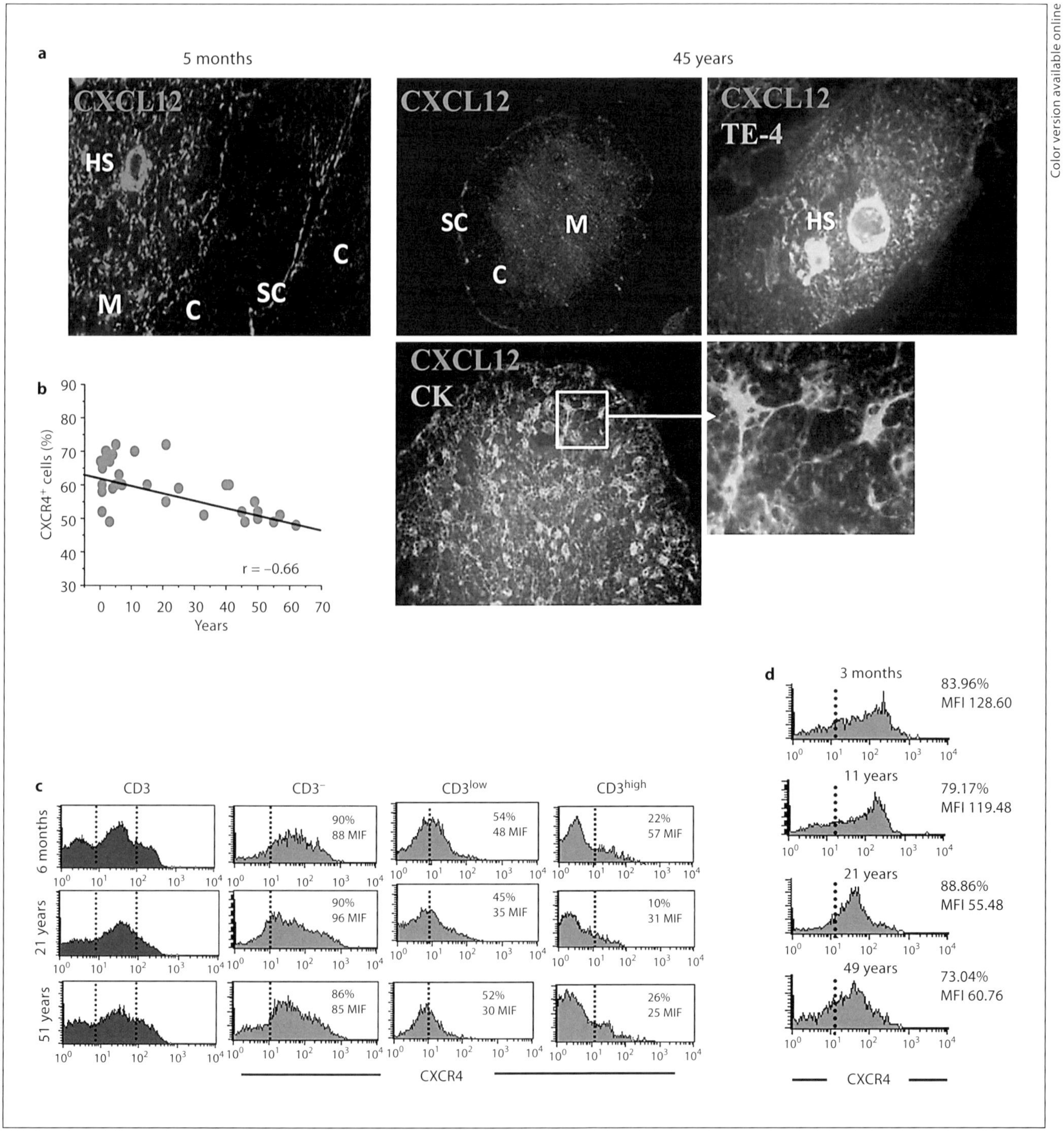

Fig. 1. Expression of CXCL12 and CXCR4 in the aged human thymus. **a** Immunohistochemical detection of CXCL12 in the subcapsule (SC) and medulla (M). Note the association of CXCL12 staining with keratin (CK)-positive TEC. HS = Hassall's bodies; C = thymic cortex. **b** Proportions of total thymic CXCR4+ cells in human thymuses of different ages. **c** CXCR4 expression in thymocyte subsets defined by CD3 expression. **d** Decreased numbers of CXCR4 on the surface of CD34+ thymic cells during aging. MFI = Mean fluorescence intensity.

CXCR4 Expression in the Thymus of Aged Humans

No significant variations were observed in the proportions of thymic CXCR4$^+$ cells in older thymuses. The percentage of CXCR4$^+$ cells in older thymuses was in the range described in the younger ones, although their values were in the lower level of such range in samples from individuals older than 20 years (fig. 1b).

As previously demonstrated [4] in young thymuses, most CD3$^-$ thymocytes expressed CXCR4 (around 90%) and the proportion of CXCR4$^+$ cells gradually decreased in CD3^{low} thymocytes that largely included the DP cells (around 50%) and CD3^{hi} SP and DP thymocytes (around 20%). However, in each of these cell subpopulations the proportion of CXCR4$^+$ cells remained basically unaltered when younger and older samples were comparatively evaluated (fig. 1c). Thus, the percentage of CXCR4-expressing CD34$^+$ cells did not changed throughout the life, but from the second decade of life onward, there was a significant reduction in the mean fluorescence intensity (MFI) of CXCR4 molecule (fig. 1d). On the contrary, the CD127 (IL-7 receptor α chain) expression on CD34$^+$ thymocytes did not change during aging (data not shown), although a reduced production of IL-7 with age has been reported [8].

Conclusions

These results demonstrate no important alterations in the expression of both CXCL12 and CXCR4 in the human thymus during aging, suggesting that as in younger thymuses, these molecules could play a role in the control of thymus homeostasis during aging. On the other hand, the lower numbers of receptors expressed by CD34$^+$ lymphoid progenitors in older respect to younger thymuses together with the difficulties to establish direct correlations between the expression of CXCL12/CXCR4 and that of the IL-7/IL-7R pair, as reported in younger thymuses [4] could explain partially the low numbers known to occur in the aged thymuses, although they maintain unchanged proportions of CD4/CD8 thymocyte subsets. More functional studies are necessary, however, to confirm whether CXCL12 is involved also in aged thymuses in the control of the survival of CD34$^+$ lymphoid progenitors and other thymocyte subsets, as observed in younger ones.

References

1 Li M, Ransohoff RM: Multiple roles of chemokine CXCL12 in the central nervous system: a migration from immunology to neurobiology. Prog Neurobiol 2008;84:116–131.
2 Klein RS, Rubin JB: Immune and nervous system CXCL12 and CXCR4: parallel roles in patterning and plasticity. Trends Immunol 2004;25:306–314.
3 Lucas D, Battista M, Shi PA, Isola L, Frenette PS: Mobilized hematopoietic stem cell yield depends on species-specific circadian timing. Cell Stem Cell 2008;3:364–366.
4 Hernandez-Lopez C, Varas A, Sacedon R, Jimenez E, Munoz JJ, Zapata AG, Vicente A: Stromal cell-derived factor 1/CXCR4 signaling is critical for early human T-cell development. Blood 2002;99:546–554.
5 Hernandez-Lopez C, Valencia J, Hidalgo L, Martinez VG, Zapata AG, Sacedon R, Varas A, Vicente A: CXCL12/CXCR4 signaling promotes human thymic dendritic cell survival regulating the Bcl-2/Bax ratio. Immunol Lett 2008;120:72–78.
6 Aw D, Taylor-Brown F, Cooper K, Palmer DB: Phenotypical and morphological changes in the thymic microenvironment from ageing mice. Biogerontology 2009;10:311–322.
7 Gui J, Zhu X, Dohkan J, Cheng L, Barnes PF, Su DM: The aged thymus shows normal recruitment of lymphohematopoietic progenitors but has defects in thymic epithelial cells. Int Immunol 2007;19:1201–1211.
8 Aspinall R, Andrew D: Thymic atrophy in the mouse is a soluble problem of the thymic environment. Vaccine 2000;18:1629–1637.

Author Index Vol. 17, No. 3, 2010

KARGER

Fax +41 61 306 12 34
E-Mail karger@karger.ch
www.karger.com

Accessible online at:
www.karger.com/nim

Subject Index Vol. 17, No. 3, 2010

KARGER

Fax +41 61 306 12 34
E-Mail karger@karger.ch
www.karger.com

Accessible online at:
www.karger.com/nim